D0365662

ATLAS OF ORAL PATHOLOGY

This atlas, either the whole or any of its parts, can also be used to obtain continuing education credits. For further details, contact the Division of Continuing Dental Education, School of Dentistry, University of Minnesota, Health Sciences Unit A6-406, 515 Delaware Street S.E., Minneapolis, Minnesota 55455.

Publication of this book was assisted by a McKnight Foundation grant to the University of Minnesota Press's program in the health sciences.

Atlas of
Oral Pathology

William G. Young, B.D.S., M.Sc., F.R.C.D.(C)
University of Queensland
Brisbane, Australia

Heddie O. Sedano, D.D.S., Dr. O
University of Minnesota School of Dentistry
Minneapolis, Minnesota

University of Minnesota Press
Minneapolis

Copyright © 1981 by the University of Minnesota.
All rights reserved.
Published by the University of Minnesota Press,
2037 University Avenue Southeast, Minneapolis, MN 55414
Printed in the United States of America.

Library of Congress Cataloging in Publication Data

Young, William G
    Atlas of oral pathology.

    Includes index.
      1. Teeth — Diseases — Atlases. 2. Mouth — Diseases
— Atlases. 3. Teeth — Diseases — Case studies.
4. Mouth — Diseases — Case studies. I. Sedano, Heddie O.,
joint author. II. Title [DNLM: 1. Mouth diseases —
Atlases. 2. Dentistry — Atlases. WU 17 Y78a]
RK287.Y68   617'.52207   80-29439
ISBN 0-8166-1040-1

The University of Minnesota
is an equal-opportunity
educator and employer.

Contents

Foreword

This most welcome aid to dentists, physicians, and other health science professionals fills a void that has existed for a long time. It represents the distillation of almost 40 years of aggregate clinical and microscopic experience in the field of oral pathology. The authors are to be praised for their effort, encompassing long hours, in choosing just the right transparency to illustrate the condition. They are superb teachers, and their skill is reflected in this atlas.

There is something in this manual for everyone—from the tyro to the expert who merely wishes to flex his or her diagnostic muscles. The format of the atlas provides ample latitude to treat the material as a detective would treat evidence in solving a case. It can and should be fun as well as purely educational. In that the authors have succeeded. I hope the reader will enjoy the atlas as much as I have.

Robert J. Gorlin

Preface

This atlas is designed to give dentists, physicians, and other health science professionals access to a large selection of cases illustrating oral pathology. It can be used in reviewing clinical oral pathology for licensing board examinations, in obtaining continuing education credits, or in identifying diseases in the clinic.

The first part of the book is divided into five chapters. Chapter 1 covers pathology of the face and neck; chapter 2 deals with pathology of the buccal mucosa, the tongue, and the floor of the mouth; and chapter 3 is concerned with pathology of the gingiva and the palate. Chapter 4 considers pathology of the teeth themselves, whereas chapter 5 handles pathology of the bone. Each of these chapters is accompanied by a microfiche illustrating the clinical and radiographic presentation of most diseases that occur in the mouth and adjacent tissues. Each chapter is divided into three sections. First, patient histories are provided. Then, a differential diagnosis is presented for each of the cases. Last, the final diagnosis for each case is given.

The second part of the book consists of a short description of each disease presented in the microfiches including its etiologic agent, clinical features, differential diagnosis, laboratory aids, and indications for treatment. The descriptions are arranged in alphabetical order according to the substantive name of the condition. Thus, acute cellulitis is alphabetized under *C*, whereas traumatic bone cyst is alphabetized under *T*.

The final part of the book consists of a cross-index for both microfiche and theory. Throughout the book, numbers assigned to the cases correspond to those of the illustrations as given on the microfiches.

This organization allows the atlas to be used in several ways. Students who wish to test their knowledge of oral pathology should read the history in the first section and view the corresponding clinical photograph or radiograph on the microfiche. They should then draw up a differential diagnosis. If they are unable to do so, they can use the differential diagnosis section as a multiple-choice item, choosing what they consider to be the best diagnosis and comparing their choice with the final diagnosis given in the third section.

To use the atlas as a standard textbook or to find illustrations of a particular disease, the student should consult the index. This gives the coordinates of the frames on the fiche or fiches that illustrate that disease, and refers to the short description of the disease in Part 2.

The histories given are of the type usually allowed in licensing examinations. They are short and incomplete but contain the information essential for a good differential diagnosis. The differential diagnoses will help students consider more diseases and general syndromes with which they may be unfamiliar. The best clinician is often the one who can think of the most possibilities and select from among them the most probable. However, because of the limitations of clinical diagnosis, a short list of about three to five diagnoses is often as far as the best clinician can go without access to further information or the results of a biopsy or laboratory tests. Accordingly, we offer approximately this number, in alphabetical order, unless the diagnosis is extremely obvious. It has not been possible to include an explanation of how the final diagnoses were made. In some cases, the diagnosis is apparent from the information given; in others, it is the result of further data from the patient, from the progress of the disease, with or without treatment, or from the laboratory.

The terminology used in the differential and final diagnoses requires some explanation. The terms "malignant neoplasm" and "infection" are often too general for inclusion in a differential diagnosis. In each case history, the site and the tissue involved should allow for more precision, so the terms "lymphoma" and "lymphadenitis" will be used. However, "Hodgkin's lymphoma" and "tuberculous lymphadenitis" would be too precise without histologic data. Consequently, the terminology used in the final diagnosis may be considerably more specific than that used in the differential diagnosis. Similarly, the term "leukoplakia" is used in the differential diagnosis as a clinical term to signify an adherent white patch, and the final diagnosis is qualified on the basis of histologic data.

For standard terminology we have, in general, used the third edition of W. G. Shafer, M. K. Hine, and B. M. Levy's *Textbook of Oral Pathology* (Philadelphia: W. B. Saunders, 1974) as our reference, with the synonyms and eponyms following the term they use in parentheses. The disadvantages of eponyms are well known, but their unfortunate prevalence in examinations necessitates their inclusion here.

The selection of diseases has been dictated by their frequency of occurrence, by their importance as life-threatening or inherited conditions, by the likelihood of their appearance on examinations, and to a lesser degree by the need to illustrate conditions of great similarity. (Similar conditions have been grouped in the

PREFACE

microfiches so that they can be contrasted.) Of greatest importance, however, has been the inclusion of neoplasms and severe systemic diseases with oral manifestations that the dentist must recognize during examination and care of the patient. It is the evaluation of this competence that necessitates the inclusion of clinical oral pathology in most licensure examinations throughout the world.

Acknowledgments

The authors wish to express their appreciation to Dr. Robert J. Gorlin for his encouragement in preparing this book, Dr. Robert S. Edmunds for his aid in preparing and selecting the photographs, Mr. LeRoy Christenson and his staff for their invaluable help in processing the photographic material, Ms. Susan Schwarze and Ms. A. J. Stephenson for their patient and careful typing, Ms. Virginia Hansen for her proofreading of the typescript, and Ms. Ann Seivert for her copy editing of the final manuscript.

The production of the five microfiches was made possible by Educational Development Grant #0-114-1914 from the University of Minnesota.

PART 1 CLINICAL ORAL PATHOLOGY CASES

CHAPTER 1

Face and Neck

Before you read the patient histories, consult the preface for directions on how to use this atlas.

Patient Histories

1A1 and 1A2
This 13-year-old male patient was born with this facial appearance. No other member of his family had similar facies. He was slightly mentally retarded.

1A3, 1A4, and 1A5
A woman 18 years old had these congenital alterations of her face, hands, feet, and mouth. There was no family history of such a condition.

1A6
This 14-year-old girl was born with this facial appearance. The patient was deaf. No other member of her family was so affected.

1A7
This facial condition had appeared overnight in a 20-year-old woman. She had been exposed to cold wind while skiing the previous day.

1A8 and 1A9
A 33-year-old woman had had this condition since birth. Two attempts at surgical correction were unsuccessful, resulting in facial palsy.

1A10
This 53-year-old man had developed these facial lesions progressively throughout his life. Some brown-pigmented patches were seen on his skin. He had several lumps on his tongue. His daughter was similarly affected.

1A11
A 58-year-old man had had pigmented lesions on his face since age 12. Some of these had been removed. In addition, he had multiple cysts of the mandible and two bifid ribs. His son and his uncle were similarly affected.

3

1A12

A 36-year-old white man had noticed this lesion 2 or 3 years ago. Since that time it had approximately doubled in size, and it tended to bleed on being scraped.

1B13

The facial lesions of this 29-year-old woman had been present for the last 4 days. Similar lesions were observed on her trunk and hands. Intraorally, she had three silvery white lesions on the buccal mucosa. She related a vague history of a lump on her lip that had healed without treatment, 7 months ago.

1B14 and 1B15

A 5-year-old girl developed a fever and this rash over a period of 3 days. Similar lesions were observed on her skin and inside her mouth. The skin lesions on her arm are also illustrated.

1B16, 1B17, and 1B18

The skin lesions on this 4-year-old girl developed over a period of 4 days. She was febrile and markedly tired, and had photophobia. Three sites are illustrated.

1B19

This facial deformity was observed in a newborn infant. There was no family history of similarly affected persons.

1B20

This 13-year-old boy had no history of allergies or other systemic diseases. His parents said that he was born with thick lips and puffy eyelids.

1B21

This 18-year-old man had had enlarged and painful lips for 3 months. He did not have scrotal tongue or facial paralysis.

1B22

A 30-year-old man had an edematous swelling of the lower lip that had been present for 2 days. The patient was under treatment for rheumatic fever.

1B23

The lip lesion on this 24-year-old man was first noticed 2 hours after dental treatment.

1B24

A 24-year-old woman had had this lesion for 2 days. A similar lesion was observed on the border of the tongue. She had a history of repeated intraoral ulceration and had used silver nitrate, recommended by her dentist, to treat a lingual aphthous ulcer.

1C25

The mother of this 5-year-old girl was concerned about her child's facial appearance. The child had complained lately of itching in the affected area.

1C26

A 9-year-old girl had had these lip lesions since birth. In addition, she had a cleft palate. The patient's father and a brother had identical clinical findings.

1C27

A 14-year-old girl had these skin markings, which had been present since birth. The patient's mother gave a vague history of "infectious disease" while pregnant with the patient. In addition, the patient had some hearing loss and wore thick eyeglasses.

1C28

This 65-year-old woman had a solitary pigmented lesion on her lower lip that had been present for several years without increasing in size.

1C29

A 48-year-old man had had these lip lesions since birth. As he had aged they had tended to fade. He had had occasional intestinal upsets. His two sons presented identical lip lesions.

1C30

A 60-year-old woman had these lesions on her lips and similar lesions on the buccal mucosa, the skin of the face, and the ears. The patient had had repeated nasal hemorrhage. Her mother and a brother had been similarly affected.

1C31

A 65-year-old woman developed the present lesion on a preexisting vesicular eruption. The patient had a slight fever, and she had been exposed to a child with chicken pox.

1C32

This 22-year-old man had been troubled by skin problems all his life. His complaint was an oral burning sensation, especially at the corners of his mouth. He also had lesions on his eyes, on his forehead, and in his groin. Skin tests to various antigens were nonreactive.

1C33

A 55-year-old edentulous man complained of burning and itching sensations at the commissure of the lip. The patient had loss of vertical dimension from prolonged denture wearing.

1C34

The lesion in this 26-year-old man evolved in 2 days and was accompanied by a burning sensation and slight discomfort. He had had similar episodes in about the same location.

1C35

A 48-year-old man had had this painless lesion for 4 days. It had indurated borders. Several painless, easily movable cervical lymph nodes were palpable.

1C36

This 50-year-old man, who was a chronic pipe smoker, had this painless and slowly progressive ulceration on his lower lip. It had been present for a year. There was no clinical evidence of regional lymph node involvement.

1D37

An 86-year-old white fisherman had noticed a painless whitening of his lower lip at least 3 years ago. It was slightly ulcerated.

1D38

A 52-year-old woman had developed these lip and skin lesions over the last 2 months. There were similar lesions on other areas of her skin, especially on the forearms. The patient stated that she felt slightly tired; however, the result of a hemoglobin estimation was within normal limits. The patient also had a history of arthritis.

1D39

A 55-year-old man had had a white patch on his lower lip for 2 years. The lesion was painless and could not be rubbed off.

1D40

This 59-year-old man said that the present lesion had grown rapidly over the last two months. It was slightly painful and on palpation it was noted to be firm. A firm lymph node was palpated in the right cervical chain.

1D41

A 15-year-old girl presented with a painless white lesion on her right commissure.

1D42

A 56-year-old woman complained of a sore on her cheek with swelling and discharge. A radiograph showed distal caries in the maxillary cuspid and periapical radiolucency at the apex of that tooth.

1D43

A 70-year-old male farmer presented with this painful and draining lesion on his right cheek. Discharging sinuses were also present in his knee. He related symptoms of an upper respiratory tract infection a month ago, accompanied by weight loss. No teeth were involved.

1D44 and 1D45

A 68-year-old woman presented with discharge from the central portion of her chin. She said it had been present for more than 4 months and that it had started with pain and swelling. The X ray of the anterior mandibular teeth is also shown.

1D46

A 59-year-old man developed a hard, slowly growing mass beneath his lower jaw 2 weeks after the extraction of a mandibular molar. The discharge from the lesion contained some yellow granules.

1D47

A 33-year-old woman of North American Indian descent had swelling of her cervical lymph nodes and abscesses in her neck that perforated and discharged. Acid-fast bacilli were recovered from the exudate.

1D48

A 44-year-old woman had had this submandibular mass for the last 3 months with episodes of enlargement and reduction in size. It was hard on palpation and fixed to deeper structures. There was no intraoral pathology. The patient's general health was apparently good.

1E49

This 63-year-old woman, a Vietnamese refugee, had had this swelling below her ear for 2 months. It was semihard and easily movable. The patient had vitiligo but otherwise was apparently in good health.

1E50

A 78-year-old woman had a firm, tender swelling behind the angle of the mandible and a complaint of soreness and pain of 2 days' duration. Saliva containing pus could be expressed from Stensen's duct. There was a history of influenza, 4 weeks ago.

1E51

A 62-year-old woman complained of a progressive enlargement below the mandibular angle over the last 4 years. The mass was painless and was fluctant on palpation. Salivary flow on the affected side was diminished.

1E52

A 49-year-old man had this neck mass, which had been growing slowly over the last 4 years. It was semisolid on palpation, easily movable, and painless. The patient was otherwise in good health.

1E53

A 31-year-old man complained of a progressive enlargement in the left side of his neck for a year. The mass was fluctuant and painless on palpation.

1E54

This 6-year-old boy was seen with a marked swelling at the angle of the mandible. According to his mother, the lesion was originally small but had grown steadily since birth. The mass was fluctuant, painless, and pulsating. The child was otherwise healthy.

1E55

A 2-year-old girl had had this neck mass from birth without a change in its size. It was painless and fluctuant.

1E56

A 6-year-old boy had a marked swelling of the left submandibular area. According to his parents, this had started growing a week ago. On palpation it was fluctuant and slightly painful. The floor of the mouth was raised. The child was otherwise in good health.

1E57

This 31-year-old woman complained of a painful marked submental enlargement over the last 3 days. She related similar previous episodes.

1E58

A 24-year-old woman had this midline enlargement of the neck for the last month. It was slightly painful and semisolid on palpation.

1E59

This 22-year-old woman complained of a submental mass of approximately 2 weeks' duration. It was tender on palpation and easily movable. There were no other cervical masses palpable.

1E60

A 24-year-old woman complained of a tender lump of 30 days' duration over the body of the mandible just anterior to the insertion of the masseter. The lump was about 1 cm in diameter and was freely movable and moderately firm. No dental cause was found.

Differential Diagnoses

1A1 and 1A2

Acrocephalosyndactyly (Apert's syndrome)

Craniofacial dysostosis (Crouzon's syndrome)

1A3, 1A4, and 1A5

Acrocephalosyndactyly (Apert's
  syndrome)
Craniofacial dysostosis (Crouzon's
  syndrome)

1A6

Cleft palate, micrognathia, and
  glossoptosis (Pierre Robin's
  anomalad)
Mandibulofacial dysostosis (Treacher
  Collins's syndrome)
Micrognathia

1A7

Auriculotemporal syndrome (Frey's
  syndrome)
Bell's palsy
Jaw-winking syndrome
Melkersson-Rosenthal's syndrome

1A8 and 1A9

Encephalofacial angiomatosis
  (Sturge-Weber's syndrome)
Melkersson-Rosenthal's syndrome
Neurofibromatosis of
  von Recklinghausen

1A10

Multiple hamartoma and neoplasia
  syndrome (Cowden's syndrome)
Neurofibromatosis of
  von Recklinghausen
Osteomatosis and intestinal polyposis
  syndrome (Gardner's syndrome)
Tuberosclerosis
Turban tumors

1A11

Multiple basal cell carcinomas
Multiple nevoid basal cell carcinoma
  syndrome (Gorlin's syndrome)

1A12

Basal cell epithelioma (basal cell carcinoma)

Malignant melanoma
  (melanocarcinoma)
Sebaceous cyst
Xanthelasma (xanthomatosis)

1B13

Acne vulgaris
Lupus erythematosus
Secondary syphilis

1B14 and 1B15

Chicken pox (varicella)
Erythema multiforme
Impetigo
Kaposi's varicelliform eruption
Rubella (German measles)

1B16, 1B17, and 1B18

Chicken pox (varicella)
Erythema multiforme
Kaposi's varicelliform eruption
Rubella (German measles)

1B19

Isolated cleft lip
Isolated cleft lip and palate
Trisomy 13

1B20

Cheilitis granulomatosa (Miescher's
  syndrome)
Double lip, blepharochalasis, and
  nontoxic thyroid enlargement
  (Ascher's syndrome)
Lymphangioma
Melkersson-Rosenthal's syndrome

1B21

Actinic cheilitis
Angioedema (angioneurotic edema)
Cheilitis glandularis
Cheilitis granulomatosa (Miescher's
  syndrome)

1B22

Angioedema (angioneurotic edema)
Lymphangioma
Melkersson-Rosenthal's syndrome

1B23

Angioedema (angioneurotic edema)
Hematoma
Traumatic ulceration

1B24

Chemical burn
Lichen planus
Lupus erythematosus
Secondary syphilis (mucous patch)

1C25

Child abuse (battered child syndrome)
Erysipelas
Lip licking
Trauma

1C26

Cleft lip/palate and congenital lip pits
  syndrome
Congenital lip pits
Mucous retention phenomenon
  (mucoceles)
Trauma

1C27

Chronic cheilitis
Congenital syphilis (rhagades)
Premature skin aging
Variation of skin creases

1C28

Ephelis
Lentigo maligna melanoma
Nevus
Tattoo

1C29

Diffuse melanosis
Hereditary intestinal polyposis
  syndrome (Peutz-Jeghers's
  syndrome)
Multiple freckles

1C30

Angiokeratoma corporis diffusum
  (Fabry's syndrome)
Blood dyscrasia
Hereditary hemorrhagic telangiectasia
  (Osler-Rendu-Weber's syndrome)
Multiple petechiae
Varicosities

1C31

Erythema multiforme
Herpes zoster (shingles)
Primary herpes simplex with
  secondary infection

1C32

Angioedema (angioneurotic edema)
Endocrine-candidiasis syndrome
Mucocutaneous candidiasis
  (moniliasis)

1C33

Angular cheilitis (perlèche)
Commissural lip pits
Trauma

1C34

Chancre
Recurrent herpes simplex (herpes
  labialis)
Squamous cell carcinoma
Trauma

1C35

Primary syphilis (chancre)
Recurrent herpes simplex (herpes
  labialis)
Squamous cell carcinoma
Trauma

1C36

Keratoacanthoma
Primary syphilis (chancre)
Squamous cell carcinoma
Traumatic ulceration

1D37

Candidiasis (moniliasis)
Chronic actinic cheilitis (solar
  keratosis)
Leukoplakia
Squamous cell carcinoma

1D38

Allergic reaction
Lichen planus
Lupus erythematosus
Primary tuberculosis (lupus vulgaris)

1D39

Chemical burn
Leukoplakia
Lichen planus
Squamous cell carcinoma

1D40

Basal cell carcinoma
Keratoacanthoma
Squamous cell carcinoma
Tuberculous ulceration

1D41

Keratoacanthoma
Papilloma
Verruca vulgaris (wart)

1D42

Acne vulgaris
Actinomycosis
Dental sinus
Primary tuberculosis (lupus vulgaris)

1D43

Actinomycosis
Basal cell carcinoma
Blastomycosis
Osteomyelitis

1D44 and 1D45

Actinomycosis

Osteomyelitis
Periapical granuloma or cyst and dental
  sinus

1D46

Actinomycosis
Anthrax
Blastomycosis
Osteomyelitis

1D47

Actinomycosis
Cat-scratch disease
Tuberculous lymphadenitis (scrofula)

1D48

Branchial cleft cyst
Chronic sialadenitis
Lymphadenitis
Lymphoma
Metastasis to lymph node

1E49

Branchial cleft cyst
Lymphadenitis
Lymphoma
Pleomorphic adenoma (mixed tumor)
Tuberculous lymphadenitis

1E50

Acute parotitis
Salivary gland neoplasm
Sialolithiasis
Sjögren's syndrome

1E51

Branchial cleft cyst
Parotid gland cyst
Parotid neoplasm

1E52

Branchial cleft cyst
Carotid body tumor
Lymphadenitis
Parotid cyst
Parotid neoplasm

1E53

Branchial cleft cyst
Carotid body tumor
Hemangioma
Hydatid cyst

1E54

Branchial cleft cyst
Cystic hygroma
Lymphoma
Parotid neoplasm

1E55

Branchial cleft cyst
Cystic hygroma
Juvenile hemangioma

1E56

Chronic or acute abscess
Hemangioma
Lymphangioma
Ranula

1E57

Dermoid cyst
Epidermoid cyst
Sialadenitis
Thyroglossal tract cyst

1E58

Dermoid cyst
Epidermoid cyst
Thyroglossal tract cyst
Thyroid neoplasm

1E59

Dermoid cyst
Epidermoid cyst
Lymphadenitis
Lymphoepithelial cyst
Ranula

1E60

Abscess
Epidermoid cyst
Nonspecific lymphadenitis

Final Diagnoses

1A1 and 1A2
Craniofacial dysotosis (Crouzon's syndrome) (p. 104)

1A3, 1A4, and 1A5
Acrocephalosyndactyly (Apert's syndrome) (p. 79)

1A6
Mandibulofacial dysostosis (Treacher Collin's syndrome) (p. 158)

1A7
Bell's palsy (p. 83)

1A8 and 1A9
Encephalofacial angiomatosis (Sturge-Weber's syndrome) (p. 200)

1A10
Neurofibromatosis of von Recklinghausen (p. 168)

1A11
Multiple nevoid basal cell carcinoma syndrome (Gorlin's syndrome) (p. 165)

1A12
Basal cell epithelioma (basal cell carcinoma) (p. 82)

1B13
Secondary syphilis (p. 201)

1B14 and 1B15
Chicken pox (varicella) (p. 98)

1B16, 1B17, and 1B18
Erythema multiforme (p. 116)

1B19
Isolated cleft lip and palate (p. 99)

1B20
Double lip, blepharochalasis, and nontoxic thyroid enlargement (Ascher's syndrome) (p. 80)

1B21
Cheilitis glandularis (p. 96)

1B22
Angioedema (angioneurotic edema) (p. 78)

1B23
Traumatic ulceration: lip bite under local anesthesia (p. 210)

1B24
Chemical burn: due to silver nitrate (p. 96)

1C25
Lip licking: secondarily infected with *Candida albicans* (p. 152)

1C26
Cleft lip-palate and congenital lip pits syndrome (p. 100)

1C27
Congenital syphilis (rhagades) (p. 201)

1C28
Ephelis (p. 114)

1C29
Hereditary intestinal polyposis syndrome (Peutz-Jeghers's syndrome) (p. 187)

1C30
Hereditary hemorrhagic telangiectasia (Osler-Rendu-Weber's syndrome) (p. 138)

1C31
Primary herpes simplex with secondary infection (p. 141)

1C32
Mucocutaneous candidiasis (moniliasis) (p. 89)

1C33

Angular cheilitis (perlèche) (p. 94)

1C34

Recurrent herpes simplex (herpes labialis) (p. 142)

1C35

Primary syphilis (chancre) (p. 201)

1C36

Squamous cell carcinoma (p. 198)

1D37

Chronic actinic cheilitis (solar keratosis) (p. 95)

1D38

Lupus erythematosus (p. 152)

1D39

Leukoplakia: epithelial dysplasia without invasion (p. 145)

1D40

Squamous cell carcinoma (p. 198)

1D41

Verruca vulgaris (wart) (p. 210)

1D42

Dental sinus (p. 107)

1D43

Blastomycosis: North American (p. 86)

1D44 and 1D45

Periapical granuloma and dental sinus (pp. 107, 186)

1D46

Actinomycosis (p. 65)

1D47

Tuberculous lymphadenitis (scrofula) (p. 208)

1D48

Metastasis to cervical lymph node: squamous cell carcinoma (p. 161)

1E49

Tuberculous lymphadenitis (p. 208)

1E50

Acute parotitis: possibly secondary to influenza (p. 182)

1E51

Parotid gland cyst (p. 181)

1E52

Parotid neoplasm: pleomorphic adenoma (p. 188)

1E53

Branchial cleft cyst (p. 86)

1E54

Parotid neoplasm: juvenile hemangioma (p. 137)

1E55

Cystic hygroma (p. 105)

1E56

Ranula (p. 193)

1E57

Sialadenitis: with sialolithiasis (p. 197)

1E58

Thyroglossal tract cyst (p. 205)

1E59

Lymphadenitis: secondary to acne vulgaris (p. 154)

1E60

Nonspecific lymphadenitis: facial node (p. 154)

CHAPTER 2

Buccal Mucosa, Tongue, and Floor of the Mouth

Before you read the patient histories, consult the preface for directions on how to use this atlas.

Patient Histories

2A1

This 25-year-old woman had a history of congenital enlargement of her upper lip. At 2 and 6 years of age she underwent surgery for this condition. She now has multiple, asymptomatic, translucent, and compressible lesions.

2A2

A 56-year-old man had had an accident that fractured several teeth. He complained of pain and swelling of his upper lip. Pus was expressed from the lesion.

2A3 and 2A4

This 45-year-old woman, with no symptoms, had a congenital hemangioma of the upper lip treated with radiotherapy at age 4. A radiograph of the area is also shown.

2A5

This 21-year-old woman said this lesion has been coming and going for about a month.

2A6

This 15-year-old girl had multiple intraoral lesions, predominantly located on the labial mucosa. The patient reported similar previous episodes. There was no fever or other systemic symptomatology.

2A7

This 30-year-old man had multiple large painful ulcerations on the buccal mucosa, the floor of the mouth, and the tongue. He related previous sporadic episodes of this condition over the last 4 years.

15

2A8

This 65-year-old man related a 1-month history of ulceration of the lower lip. The patient was a heavy pipe smoker. The lesion was slightly indurated on palpation. No cervical or submandibular nodes were detected on clinical inspection.

2A9

This 32-year-old woman reported intraoral bleeding of about 3 weeks' duration. The patient had been diagnosed elsewhere as having acute necrotizing ulcerative gingivitis and had been treated accordingly, with no success. The patient felt slightly dizzy and was pale.

2A10

This 33-year-old white man had first noticed these lesions 3 years ago. The patient's history revealed gastrointestinal problems from regional enteritis. The patient was on prednisone therapy.

2A11

This 20-year-old girl had slightly painful red areas on her tongue and cheek that had lasted approximately a month and then regressed.

2A12

This 50-year-old woman complained of bleeding, upon minimal trauma, from this lesion, which had been present for a long time.

2B13

This 71-year-old edentulous woman stated that the present lesion had appeared overnight. She vaguely recalled a similar episode a few months earlier. The patient was otherwise in good health.

2B14

The lesions on this 26-year-old woman were discovered by a dental student on routine examination. There were no systemic signs or symptoms. The patient was in good health.

2B15

This 18-year-old girl had had pain, slight swelling distal to the lower left second molar, and difficulty in opening her mouth, for 3 days. She had attempted to relieve the pain.

2B16

This 33-year-old woman was extremely concerned because she had been told by her dentist a week earlier that this bilateral condition in her mouth was precancerous and dangerous.

2B17

This 10-year-old girl had white plaquelike lesions resembling milk curds that could be stripped off, leaving bleeding areas.

2B18

Both cheeks, the lips and the tongue mucosae of this 17-year-old boy had been dull white for at least 3 months. The coating, when removed, left a rough, non-bleeding surface. His father and father's cousin were similarly affected.

2B19

This 23-year-old woman complained of a metallic taste. The buccal mucosal lesions had been present for 3 days. There was no skin involvement. The remainder of the oral mucosa was normal.

2B20

This 24-year-old man had used snuff since age 18.

2B21

This 50-year-old man was a heavy pipe smoker.

2B22

This 54-year-old man had a long history of snuff use. The present lesion was tender and had an indurated base. The teeth in the area had rough edges.

2B23

This 78-year-old white man had first noticed this lesion 6 months earlier when he slipped and bruised his face. The lesion was painful and had been so for 3 weeks, especially on chewing. His physician had referred to the lesion as a "canker sore."

2B24

A 35-year-old woman had a painful ulceration at the level of the occlusal plane. The patient admitted to cheek and lip chewing.

2C25

This 50-year-old man had yellowish spots located bilaterally on the mucosa of both cheeks. They were asymptomatic and had been present almost all his life.

2C26

This 78-year-old edentulous white man had a hard, painless nodule on the buccal mucosa that was radiopaque on X-ray examination. The lump had been present for some time and had swollen up and burst 2 months ago.

2C27

This 32-year-old woman had a circumscribed, slow-growing, painless white lesion on her cheek.

2C28

A 48-year-old man had an asymptomatic, slow-growing, and easily movable mass on the floor of the mouth. Cheesy material was expressed from the lesion.

2C29 and 2C30

A 28-year-old man had a slowly enlarging mass on the floor of the mouth, painful during mastication. A radiograph of the area is also shown.

2C31

An 8-year-old boy had a slowly enlarging, unilateral, painless, and fluctuant mass in the floor of the mouth.

2C32

A 25-year-old man had a unilateral enlargement on the floor of the mouth, causing partial elevation of the tongue. It was semisolid on palpation and had been present for 3 months.

2C33

This 5-year-old girl had fallen with a pencil in her mouth. There was a slightly enlarged and painful node in the submental region.

2C34

This 64-year-old man complained of pain and inability to move his tongue properly. This lesion had been present for 2 months and had been diagnosed previously as a traumatic ulceration produced by sharp teeth. The floor of the mouth in the adjacent area was hard on palpation. A large, nontender, and firm lymph node was found in the mandibular area.

2C35

This 67-year-old woman had had these tongue lesions for a week. Several others were present on her buccal and lip mucosae. She had had many similar episodes in the past. Some areas of her oral mucosa showed scarring.

2C36

A 25-year-old woman had tongue lesions that regressed and recurred sporadically.

2D37

This 50-year-old woman had had this painful lesion on the left border of her tongue for 2 days. The lesion was not indurated and according to the patient had appeared overnight. The patient related episodes of nocturnal bruxism.

2D38

This 52-year-old woman had been complaining of glossodynia for the last 2 months, but neither her dentist nor her physician had been able to identify a cause. The present tongue appearance had developed in the course of 1 week. The involved area was hard on palpation. Tongue mobility was impaired.

2D39

A 50-year-old man had this painless lesion of approximately 3 years' duration. He smoked over a pack of cigarettes a day.

2D40

This tongue lesion was found on routine examination of a 38-year-old man. Two other similar lesions were observed on the buccal mucosa. The patient was not aware of the lesions, which were asymptomatic. Upon questioning, it was learned that the patient had a concomitant skin rash, especially over the trunk and neck. This rash had a papular erythematous appearance.

2D41

A 50-year-old man presented this tongue lesion, which had grown rapidly in the last 2 weeks. The borders were indurated and the patient complained of mild pain.

2D42

This 11-year-old girl had had this painless lesion for the last 2 years. The lesion had not increased in size.

2D43

This 50-year-old woman had had a painless lesion on the border of her tongue for a year. The lesion was freely movable and unchanging in size.

2D44

This 60-year-old man presented these elevated lesions, which, according to the patient, had appeared overnight. The patient otherwise appeared to be in good health.

2D45

A 68-year-old woman had first noticed this lesion 25 years ago. The lesion was asymptomatic and compressible.

2D46

A 65-year-old man was found to have these changes on the undersurface of his tongue.

2D47

These soft and painless lesions had been present in a 21-year-old man all his life. Similar lesions were present on the lip and the buccal mucosa.

CLINICAL ORAL PATHOLOGY CASES

2D48

These lesions were found on routine dental examination of a 22-year-old man. Similar lesions were observed in the upper lip mucosa. The patient was tall and muscularly underdeveloped. The patient stated that he had undergone thyroid surgery in order to eliminate a "tumor." The patient also had chills and night sweats of unexplained origin.

2E49

A 37-year-old white man presented for routine dental examination. The patient was unaware of the lesion. Smears were positive for *Candida albicans.*

2E50

This 3-month-old, bottle-fed infant was brought by his mother, who had noticed this lesion.

2E51

A 22-year-old man had had this tongue appearance for several years. He complained of an occasional burning sensation of his tongue.

2E52

This 42-year-old man had noticed progressive whitening of his tongue for the last 5 years. During the last 4 months, ulceration and scarring had occurred. The lesions were not painful. The patient had a positive VDRL test.

2E53

The tongue lesions of this 51-year-old woman had had a 5-year history of intermittent episodes of recurrence and remission. There was marked taste alteration and occasional pain. The patient was concerned about the possibility of having cancer.

2E54

This 40-year-old woman's tongue had presented this appearance for a year with periods of remission and exacerbation. The patient complained of a metallic taste. Two small, rounded, bluish brown, pruritic papules, of approximately the same duration, were found on her left forearm.

2E55

This 48-year-old woman complained of pain and a burning sensation in her tongue that had lasted for 2 weeks. The patient was pale and felt dizzy. She also became tired easily and had lost considerable weight during the previous month.

2E56

This 52-year-old man was referred by his dentist because of progressive enlargement of his tongue. This change had taken place over the last 8 months and was causing difficulty in swallowing. The patient was lethargic and tired easily. Multiple skin nodules of a violaceous color were found over the face, hands, and forearms. The submandibular glands were enlarged bilaterally.

2E57

This 43-year-old man stated that this condition had appeared overnight. He had been placed on a 3-week antibiotic regimen by his physician for a urinary tract infection.

2E58

This 23-year-old man had had these lesions for 2 days. Others were present on his buccal and lip mucosae. The gingiva was slightly hyperplastic, and the patient was febrile. There had been no previous episodes of similar lesions.

2E59

The tongue lesions of this 7-year-old girl had been present for 2 days. Small vesicles were observed on her hands and toes. The patient had a mildly elevated body temperature and complained of a burning sensation of her tongue. Her older brother was similarly affected.

2E60

The tip of the tongue of this 14-year-old girl reached almost to the mandibular incisors in its outermost projection. According to her mother, the patient had been born that way.

Differential Diagnoses

2A1

Focal epithelial hyperplasia
Lymphangioma
Multiple mucoceles
Multiple mucosal neuromas syndrome

2A2

Angioedema
Foreign body reaction
Salivary gland neoplasm
Sinus tract

2A3 and 2A4

Foreign body
Postradiation sarcoma
Recurrent hemangioma

2A5

Chronic sialadenitis
Lymphangioma
Mucocele
Salivary gland neoplasm

2A6

Erosive lichen planus
Major aphthous ulceration
　　(periadenitis mucosa necrotica
　　recurrens, Sutton's disease)
Minor aphthous ulceration
Primary herpetic stomatitis
Vesiculobullous disease

2A7
Cheek biting
Major aphthous ulceration
  (periadenitis mucosa necrotica
  recurrens, Sutton's disease)
Minor aphthous ulceration
Vesiculobullous disease

2A8
Leukoplakia
Secondary syphilis
Squamous cell carcinoma
Traumatic ulceration

2A9
Acute necrotizing ulcerative
  gingivostomatitis
Blood dyscrasias
Chronic hyperplastic gingivostomatitis
Erythema multiforme

2A10
Blood dyscrasia
Candidiasis (moniliasis)
Cheek biting
Drug idiosyncratic reaction
Inflammatory hyperplasia associated
  with regional enteritis (Crohn's
  disease)

2A11
Benign migratory glossitis (geographic
  tongue)
Blood dyscrasia
Drug allergies
Migratory mucositis
Self-inflicted trauma

2A12
Arteriovenous aneurysm
Hemangioma
Hematoma
Lymphangioma

2B13
Blood dyscrasia
Hemangioma
Hematoma
Malignant melanoma

2B14
Addison's disease
Amalgam tattoo
Chloroquine pigmentation
Idiopathic melanotic pigmentation
Peutz-Jegher's syndrome
Physiologic (racial) pigmentation

2B15
Aspirin burn
Leukoedema
Leukoplakia
Pericoronitis

2B16
Acute pseudomembranous candidiasis
  (moniliasis)
Leukoplakia
Lichen planus
Linea alba

2B17
Acute pseudomembranous candidiasis
  (moniliasis)
Cheek biting
Leukoedema
Leukoplakia
Lichen planus

2B18
Acute pseudomembranous candidiasis
  (moniliasis)
Cheek biting
Leukoedema
White sponge nevus (Cannon's disease)

2B19

Acute pseudomembranous candidiasis
  (moniliasis)
Cheek biting
Hyperkeratosis
Lichen planus
Lupus erythematosus

2B20

Aspirin burn
Hyperkeratosis secondary to use of
  snuff
Leukoplakia
Lichen planus

2B21

Candidiasis (moniliasis)
Hyperkeratosis secondary to smoking
Leukoplakia
Linea alba

2B22

Leukoplakia
Snuff dipper's pouch
Squamous cell carcinoma
Traumatic ulceration

2B23

Leukoplakia
Noma
Squamous cell carcinoma
Traumatic ulceration

2B24

Cheek biting
Leukoplakia
Linea alba
Squamous cell carcinoma

2C25

Fordyce's granules
Keratosis follicularis (Darier's disease)
Leukoplakia

Lichen planus
Xanthomatosis

2C26

Calcified lipoma or fibroma
Calcified lymph node
Phlebolith
Sialolith

2C27

Fibroepithelial polyp
Papilloma
Traumatic neuroma

2C28

Abscess
Dermoid cyst
Epidermoid cyst
Lymphoepithelial cyst
Ranula

2C29 and 2C30

Chronic sialadenitis
Dermoid cyst
Sialolithiasis

2C31

Dermoid cyst
Lymphoepithelial cyst
Ranula
Sialolithiasis

2C32

Acute infection or cellulitis of the floor
  of the mouth
Dermoid cyst
Salivary gland neoplasm

2C33

Aphthous ulceration
Electrical burn
Ruptured mucocele
Traumatic ulceration

2C34

Granulomatous inflammation
Salivary gland neoplasm
Squamous cell carcinoma
Traumatic ulceration

2C35

Benign mucous membrane pemphigoid
Erythema multiforme
Major aphthous ulceration
(periadenitis mucosa necrotica
recurrens, Sutton's disease)
Minor aphthous ulceration

2C36

Benign migratory glossitis (geographic
tongue)
Erosive lichen planus
Oral psoriasis
Traumatic ulceration

2D37

Benign migratory glossitis
Granulomatous ulceration
Squamous cell carcinoma
Traumatic ulceration

2D38

Malignant neoplasm
Specific granuloma (e.g., tuberculosis)
Squamous cell carcinoma

2D39

Hyperkeratosis
Leukoplakia
Moniliasis
Squamous cell carcinoma

2D40

Candidiasis (moniliasis)
Leukoplakia
Lichen planus
Lupus erythematosus
Secondary syphilis (mucous patch)

2D41

Chancre
Squamous cell carcinoma
Traumatic ulceration
Tuberculous ulceration

2D42

Ectopic lymphoid tissue
Granular cell myoblastoma
Lipoma
Neurogenic neoplasm
Traumatic fibroma

2D43

Granular cell myoblastoma
Traumatic fibroma
Traumatic neuroma

2D44

Blood dyscrasia
Hemangioma
Hematoma
Varicosity

2D45

Blood dyscrasia
Hemangioma
Hematoma
Varicosity

2D46

Hemangioma
Hematoma
Hereditary hemorrhagic telangiectasia
(Osler-Rendu-Weber's syndrome)
Lingual varicosities

2D47

Hemangiomas
Hereditary hemorrhagic telangiectasia
(Osler-Rendu-Weber's syndrome)
Lymphangiomas

2D48

Multiple lymphangiomas
Multiple mucosal neuromas, medullary
  carcinoma of the thyroid, and
  pheochromocytoma syndrome
Multiple neurilemomas
Neurofibromatosis of
  von Recklinghausen
Xanthomatosis

2E49

Early syphilitic glossitis
Hairy tongue
Lingual thyroid nodule
Median rhomboid glossitis

2E50

Candidiasis (moniliasis)
Child abuse (battered child syndrome)
Hematoma
Traumatic ulceration

2E51

Benign migratory glossitis (geographic
  tongue)
Candidiasis
Fissured tongue (scrotal tongue)

2E52

Leukoplakia
Squamous cell carcinoma
Syphilitic glossitis
Tuberculous ulceration

2E53

Erosive lichen planus
Leukoplakia
Recurrent aphthous ulcerations
Squamous cell carcinoma

2E54

Candidiasis (moniliasis)
Lichen planus
Lupus erythematosus

2E55

Anemia
Blood dyscrasia
Sjögren's syndrome
Vitamin deficiency

2E56

Amyloidosis
Lymphedema
Lymphoma (including multiple
  myeloma)

2E57

Benign migratory glossitis
Bismuth pigmentation
Black hairy tongue
Median rhomboid glossitis

2E58

Aphthous stomatitis
Erythema multiforme
Primary herpes simplex
Viral infection

2E59

Erythema multiforme
Hand-foot-and-mouth disease
Primary herpetic stomatitis

2E60

Ankyloglossia
Hyperplasia of submandibular salivary
  gland ducts
Scarring secondary to trauma

Final Diagnoses

2A1
Lymphangioma (p. 155)

2A2
Foreign body reaction: due to tooth fragments (p. 125)

2A3 and 2A4
Foreign body: Radon implant needle (p. 125)

2A5
Mucocele (p. 163)

2A6
Minor aphthous ulceration (p. 162)

2A7
Major aphthous ulceration (periadenitis mucosa necrotica recurrens, Sutton's disease) (p. 156)

2A8
Squamous cell carcinoma (p. 198)

2A9
Blood dyscrasia: acute monocytic leukemia (p. 149)

2A10
Inflammatory hyperplasia associated with regional enteritis (Crohn's disease) (p. 194)

2A11
Benign migratory glossitis with migratory mucositis (stomatitis areata migrans) (p. 84)

2A12
Hemangioma (p. 137)

2B13
Hematoma (p. 138)

2B14
Idiopathic melanotic pigmentation (p. 160)

2B15
Aspirin burn and pericoronitis (pp. 81, 186)

2B16
Linea alba (p. 151)

2B17
Acute pseudomembranous candidiasis (moniliasis) (p. 88)

2B18
White sponge nevus (Cannon's disease) (p. 213)

2B19
Lichen planus (p. 151)

2B20
Hyperkeratosis secondary to use of snuff (p. 145)

2B21
Hyperkeratosis secondary to smoking (p. 145)

2B22
Squamous cell carcinoma (p. 198)

2B23
Squamous cell carcinoma (p. 198)

2B24
Cheek biting (p. 94)

2C25
Fordyce's granules (p. 125)

2C26
Sialolith: in minor salivary gland (p. 197)

2C27

Fibroepithelial polyp (p. 118)

2C28

Lymphoepithelial cyst
(p. 155)

2C29 and 2C30

Sialolithiasis (p. 97)

2C31

Ranula (p. 193)

2C32

Dermoid cyst (p. 111)

2C33

Traumatic ulceration (p. 210)

2C34

Squamous cell carcinoma (p. 198)

2C35

Major aphthous ulceration
(periadenitis mucosa necrotica
recurrens, Sutton's disease) (p. 156)

2C36

Benign migratory glossitis (geographic
tongue) (p. 84)

2D37

Traumatic ulceration (p. 210)

2D38

Squamous cell carcinoma (p. 198)

2D39

Hyperkeratosis (p. 145)

2D40

Secondary syphilis (mucous patch)
(p. 201)

2D41

Squamous cell carcinoma (p. 198)

2D42

Granular cell myoblastoma (p. 135)

2D43

Traumatic fibroma (p. 118)

2D44

Hematoma (traumatic) (p. 138)

2D45

Hemangioma (p. 137)

2D46

Lingual varicosities (p. 151)

2D47

Lymphangiomas (p. 155)

2D48

Multiple mucosal neuromas, medullary
carcinoma of the thyroid, and
pheochromocytoma syndrome
(p. 164)

2E49

Median rhomboid glossitis (p. 158)

2E50

Traumatic ulceration: related to
suckling and acute pseudomembranous
candidiasis (pp. 88, 210)

2E51

Fissured tongue (scrotal tongue):
secondarily infected with *Candida
albicans* (pp. 122, 210)

2E52

Syphilitic glossitis (p. 201)

2E53

Erosive lichen planus (p. 151)

2E54

Lichen planus (p. 151)

CLINICAL ORAL PATHOLOGY CASES

2E55

Pernicious anemia due to vitamin B_{12} deficiency (Hunter's glossitis) (p. 211)

2E56

Amyloidosis (p. 76)

2E57

Black hairy tongue (p. 135)

2E58

Primary herpes simplex (p. 141)

2E59

Hand-foot-and-mouth disease (p. 136)

2E60

Ankyloglossia (p. 79)

CHAPTER 3

Gingiva and Palate

Before you read the patient histories, consult the preface for directions on how to use this atlas.

Patient Histories

3A1

This 11-year-old boy presented this oral appearance. The condition had been present for as long as he or his parents could remember.

3A2

This 3-day-old female infant presented with this apparently asymptomatic condition.

3A3

A 2-year-old girl presented with this circumscribed fluctuant lesion on the alveolar ridge. Her mother had noticed the lesion only a few days previously.

3A4

A female infant was born with a mass on the anterior left maxillary gingiva and alveolar ridge.

3A5

A male infant at birth was found to have a mass on the anterior left maxillary gingiva and alveolar ridge. The radiograph showed displaced tooth germs and bone destruction.

3A6

This 3-month-old infant was brought for consultation because of premature eruption of teeth. Clinical examination revealed marked mobility of the lower incisors. The surrounding gingiva was friable and bled easily. The infant also had a mild exanthema of rust color over the scalp skin. There was no history of a similarly affected individual in the family.

3A7 and 3A8

This 6-year-old girl had a history of repeated episodes of oral ulcerations affecting not only the gingiva but, on occasions, different areas of the oral mucosa. These episodes seemed to have come and gone periodically. The patient's father had similar lesions but to a lesser degree. A radiograph is also presented.

3A9, 3A10, and 3A11

This 9-year-old boy was brought for consultation because of premature exfoliation of teeth. His pantographic radiograph is also shown. The patient had very coarse palms (as shown). According to his mother, the hand condition had been present almost since birth. The patient had two apparently healthy siblings. His parents were second cousins.

3A12

This 2½-year-old girl was referred for consultation complaining of loose teeth. Her oral lesions had begun when the first primary molar became mobile. A diagnosis of diabetes insipidus had been made 4 months previously.

3B13

This 5-year-old boy presented with hyperplastic and bleeding gingivae, fever, malaise, and lassitude. Clinical examination revealed bilateral cervical lymphadenopathy.

3B14

This 19-year-old female adolescent was referred by her dentist because these gingival lesions had progressively enlarged and had not responded to conventional treatment over the previous 2 months. The patient had lost some weight and felt tired. She had chronic sinusitis and a constant cough. The patient had been complaining of bilateral pain on her flanks for the last few days. She was not taking any medication.

3B15

This 23-year-old woman had diffuse gingival enlargement and a moderate tendency for gingival bleeding. The patient was under treatment for occasional seizures.

3B16

This 42-year-old man had had these asymptomatic oral lesions for as long as he could remember. A daughter had a similar condition but to a lesser degree.

3B17

A 17-year-old male adolescent had marked gingival inflammation and painful ulcers on his lips and tongue that had been present for a few days. He complained of slight fever and pain on swallowing. Some skin lesions were also seen on his face.

3B18

This 12-year-old female adolescent had a painful and easily bleeding gingiva. She complained of an unpleasant taste and increased salivation. There were palpable, painful, bilateral, cervical lymph nodes.

3B19

This 35-year-old woman was referred by her dentist because these desquamating oral lesions had failed to heal with conventional therapy. The lesions had been present for 6 months. They had started as vesicles and after a few hours, they would break, leaving raw surfaces. The patient felt mildly tired. With the exception of a small vesicle on the skin of her face, the remainder of the skin was blister-free.

3B20

This 50-year-old man had marked halitosis, tooth mobility, and calculus. The gingival tissues were soft and edematous and bled easily.

3B21 and 3B22

A 73-year-old woman complained of discomfort in her lower left first molar. The tooth was vital but very mobile and demonstrated marked gingival recession. The remaining teeth and periodontium showed mild chronic periodontitis with calculus deposition. No systemic problems were elicited in the history.

3B23

An 18-year-old woman demonstrated this painful swelling in the area of an erupting mandibular third molar. She also complained of pain while masticating and swallowing.

3B24

This 45-year-old man complained of a "raw feeling" of about 3 months' duration. Periodontal bone loss was found radiographically on the teeth adjacent to the lesion. The patient did not smoke or drink alcohol, and he denied using snuff.

3C25

This 75-year-old man had been a snuff user for 57 years. This painful lesion had been present for 3 weeks at the site where he held the snuff.

3C26

A 76-year-old man had had this painless, pedunculated lesion for about 20 years. He was edentulous.

3C27

This 35-year-old man complained of intense pain in his right mandibular area. He related that the present lesion had evolved progressively over the last 2 months. A radiograph (not provided) of the area revealed an ill-defined, radiolucent destruction in the subjacent bone. The remainder of the clinical examination was within normal limits.

3C28

This 72-year-old man complained of loose dentures. Clinical examination revealed this painless, slow-growing lesion.

3C29

This 35-year-old woman is in the third trimester of pregnancy.

3C30

A 47-year-old woman with poor oral hygiene had first noticed this painless lesion 7 years ago. The lesion had not increased in size since that time.

3C31

A 30-year-old man had noticed this lesion a few days after extraction of the first molar. Upon radiographic examination, a small sequestrum was noticed in the tooth socket.

3C32

A 64-year-old man said that this asymptomatic lesion had "popped out" a year ago, after extraction of the maxillary canine. On clinical examination it was found to be pedunculate and to bleed easily. The patient was otherwise in good health.

3C33

A 52-year-old woman had advanced periodontal disease. This lump on her gingiva tended to bleed easily. Obstructive jaundice was also diagnosed.

3C34

A 35-year-old woman had these asymptomatic, bilateral, firm lesions, which had grown slowly for 15 years.

3C35

A 67-year-old woman had had these amalgam restorations placed 6 years ago. A fixed bridge was originally cemented over the restorations, but it had come out 2 years ago. Her general health was good.

3C36

This 50-year-old man had first noticed pigmentation of his labial and palatal gingivae 10 years ago. During this time the lesion had increased progressively in size. Two of the teeth in the area had been mobile and were extracted.

3D37

A 59-year-old man was found to have blue coloration of his palate. For many years he had swabbed his nasal passages with *Argyrol* solution for an antral infection.

3D38

This 21-year-old man had these bilateral lesions on the soft palate. They had appeared spontaneously. There was a history of epistaxis the previous week and of hepatitis in the past.

3D39

This lesion on a 28-year-old woman had appeared overnight. There was no history of any systemic disease or drug intake. The previous night the patient had had an episode of vomiting. Blood studies were ordered and they were within normal limits.

3D40

This 30-year-old woman had accidentally poked her palate with a chicken bone while eating.

3D41

This 25-year-old man complained of sore throat, nausea, and headache. Clinical examination revealed tonsillitis and bilateral, multiple cervical lymphadenitis.

3D42

A 21-year-old woman complained of malaise and increased body temperature. Apart from these lesions on the soft palate, the oral mucosa was normal. The patient did not have any dermatologic or systemic manifestations.

3D43, 3D44, and 3D45

This 65-year-old woman complained of a burning sensation in her mouth. The lesions on her palate and the erythematous areas on her gingiva resulted from vesicular lesions that had persisted for 24 hours and then ruptured. The eyes had been affected by conjunctivitis, which was followed by the development of adhesions.

3D46

A 60-year-old woman had worn the same dentures for the past 25 years. These palatal lesions were slightly painful and were accompanied by a mild burning sensation.

3D47

This 53-year-old man complained of pain and a severe burning sensation of the alveolar and palatal mucosae of 2 weeks' duration.

3D48

A 68-year-old woman who wore dentures presented with this palatal appearance and complained of a marked burning sensation and altered taste. On clinical examination several detachable white membranes were observed.

3E49

This 45-year-old man smoked more than two packages of cigarettes a day.

3E50

This 42-year-old woman smoked more than 40 cigarettes a day. A lesion similar to this one was found on the buccal mucosa of the same side.

3E51

This 35-year-old man was a reverse smoker. According to the patient, this painful lesion had been present for only a few days.

3E52

This 65-year-old woman had first noticed this asymptomatic palatal swelling 4 weeks ago. It had grown rapidly and was ill defined. Several cervical lymph nodes were enlarged; these were hard on palpation.

3E53

This 25-year-old woman had a painless swelling that had appeared 2 months ago and had slowly increased in size. It was soft on palpation.

3E54

A 30-year-old woman had severe pain and this large swelling on the palate of 2 days' duration. Clinical examination revealed a large, carious lesion on the lateral incisor as well as regional lymphadenitis.

3E55

A 62-year-old woman had this painless palatal lesion of a year's duration. It had not increased in size.

3E56

A 69-year-old woman had this bone hard palatal lesion, which had been present for a long time.

3E57

This 80-year-old man was found, on routine examination, to have this change in his soft palate. The patient had not been aware of it.

3E58

A 3-month-old female infant had had this palatal appearance since birth. She also had all of the fingers of both hands, with the exception of the thumbs, fused in a mid-digital mass.

3E59

A 17-year-old male had this appearance of his soft palate.

3E60

A woman of unstated age presented with this palatal lesion, which she said had started as a small, red, painless area a few weeks prior to consultation. It had now perforated the nasal cavity. A history of a positive serological test for syphilis several years previously was obtained.

Differential Diagnoses

3A1

Hyperplastic labial frenulum
Scarring

3A2

Enamel pearls
Exostoses
Focal epithelial hyperplasia (Heck's disease)
Fordyce's granules
Gingival cysts (Epstein's pearls, Bohn's nodules)

3A3

Eruption cyst
Gingival cyst
Hematoma
Odontogenic neoplasm

3A4

Congenital epulis of the newborn (congenital granular cell myoblastoma)
Fibrous dysplasia
Melanotic neuroectodermal tumor of infancy
Neuroblastoma
Teratoma

3A5

Congenital epulis of the newborn
Fibrous dysplasia
Melanotic neuroectodermal tumor of infancy
Neuroblastoma
Teratoma

3A6

Blood dyscrasia
Histiocytosis X
Hypophosphatasia
Neonatal teeth

3A7 and 3A8

Blood dyscrasia
Histiocytosis X
Juvenile periodontosis
Papillon-Lefèvre's syndrome
Trauma

3A9, 3A10, and 3A11

Blood dyscrasia
Hypophosphatasia
Juvenile periodontosis
Papillon-Lefèvre's syndrome

3A12

Chronic dental abscess
Histiocytosis X (Hand-Schüller-
Christian's disease)
Juvenile periodontosis
Specific granuloma

3B13

Blood dyscrasia
Fibrous hyperplasia caused by
diphenylhydantoin sodium
Gingival fibromatosis
Hyperplastic gingivitis

3B14

Blood dyscrasia
Hyperplastic gingivitis
Pyogenic granuloma
Vitamin C deficiency
Wegener's granulomatosis

3B15

Blood dyscrasia
Fibrous gingival hyperplasia caused by
diphenylhydantoin sodium
Gingival fibromatosis
Hyperplastic gingivitis

3B16

Buccal exostoses
Gingival fibromatosis
Inflammatory gingival hyperplasia

3B17

Erythema multiforme
Major aphthous ulceration
(periadenitis mucosa necrotica
recurrens, Sutton's disease)
Primary herpetic gingivostomatitis
Recurrent aphthous stomatitis

3B18

Blood dyscrasia

Primary herpetic gingivostomatitis
Recurrent necrotizing ulcerative
gingivostomatitis

3B19

Chronic desquamative gingivitis
Erosive lichen planus
Mucous membrane pemphigoid
Pemphigus vulgaris

3B20

Chronic periodontitis
Periodontal disease associated with
one of several systemic predisposing
conditions
Periodontosis
Vitamin C deficiency

3B21 and 3B22

Advanced chronic periodontitis
Eosinophilic granuloma
Histiocytosis X
Metastatic tumor
Periodontal abscess
Trauma

3B23

Mucoepidermoid tumor
Pericoronitis
Periodontal abscess

3B24

Granulomatous ulceration
Malignant primary neoplasm
Metastatic neoplasm
Periodontal disease
Traumatic ulceration

3C25

Granulomatous ulceration
Hyperkeratosis and hyperplasia
secondary to use of snuff
Leukoplakia
Squamous cell carcinoma

3C26

Papilloma
Verruca vulgaris
Verrucous carcinoma

3C27

Benign neoplasm
Malignant neoplasm
Osteomyelitis

3C28

Fibroma
Inflammatory fibrous hyperplasia
  (denture injury tumor,
  epulis fissuratum)
Squamous cell carcinoma

3C29

Blood dyscrasia
Gingival hyperplasia
Pyogenic granuloma
Trauma

3C30

Adenomatoid odontogenic tumor
Fibrous gingival hyperplasia
Peripheral giant cell granuloma
Pyogenic granuloma

3C31

Antral neoplasm
Antral polyp
Metastatic neoplasm
Pyogenic granuloma

3C32

Malignant neoplasm
Peripheral giant cell granuloma
Pyogenic granuloma

3C33

Granulomatous disease
Metastatic neoplasm

Peripheral giant cell granuloma
Pyogenic granuloma

3C34

Chondromas
Osteomas
Tori mandibularis

3C35

Amalgam tattoo
Heavy metal line
Physiologic melanotic pigmentation
  of gingiva

3C36

Amalgam tattoo
Heavy metal line
Lentigo maligna melanoma

3D37

Addison's disease
Blue nevus
Exogenous pigmentation

3D38

Blood dyscrasia
Hematoma
Vitamin K deficiency

3D39

Hematoma
Purpura
Vitamin K deficiency

3D40

Blood dyscrasia
Hemangioma
Hematoma
Vesiculobullous disease

3D41

Blood dyscrasia
Hereditary hemorrhagic telangiectasia
Infectious mononucleosis
Trauma

3D42

Hand-foot-and-mouth disease
Herpangina
Herpes simplex
Hyperplastic lymphoid aggregates
Other viral disorder

3D43, 3D44, and 3D45

Benign mucous membrane pemphigoid
Erosive lichen planus
Erythema multiforme
Pemphigus vulgaris

3D46

Candidiasis
Denture base allergy
Inflammatory papillary hyperplasia
   (palatal papillomatosis)

3D47

Denture base allergy
Denture sore mouth (denture
   stomatitis)

3D48

Atrophic candidiasis
Denture base allergy
Denture sore mouth (denture
   stomatitis)
Erosive lichen planus

3E49

Leukoplakia
Nicotinic stomatitis
Squamous cell carcinoma

3E50

Candidiasis
Leukoplakia
Lichen planus
Squamous cell carcinoma

3E51

Midline lethal granuloma

Nasal neoplasm
Noma
Squamous cell carcinoma
Tertiary syphilis (gumma)

3E52

Antral neoplasm
Bone neoplasm
Malignant lymphoma
Metastatic neoplasm
Neurofibroma

3E53

Antral neoplasm
Bone neoplasm
Cyst
Mucous retention cyst
Salivary gland neoplasm

3E54

Dentoalveolar abscess
Nasopalatine cyst
Odontogenic neoplasm
Periapical cyst

3E55

Chronic dentoalveolar abscess
Exostosis
Fibroepithelial polyp
"Fibroma"
Salivary gland neoplasm

3E56

Osteoma
Salivary gland neoplasm
Torus palatinus

3E57

Cleft palate
Midline raphae
Scar
Submucous cleft palate

3E58

Cleft palate associated with a
    chromosomal abnormality
Cleft palate associated with a syndrome
Isolated cleft palate

3E59

Bifid uvula

3E60

Improperly closed cleft palate
Midline lethal granuloma
Tertiary syphilis (gumma)

Final Diagnoses

3A1

Hyperplastic labial frenulum (p. 146)

3A2

Gingival cysts (Epstein's pearls, Bohn's nodules) (p. 132)

3A3

Eruption cyst (p. 116)

3A4

Congenital epulis of the newborn (congenital granular cell myoblastoma) (p. 102)

3A5

Melanotic neuroectodermal tumor of infancy (p. 159)

3A6

Histiocytosis X: Letterer-Siwe's disease (p. 143)

3A7 and 3A8

Blood dyscrasia: cyclic neutropenia (p. 104)

3A9, 3A10, and 3A11

Papillon-Lefèvre's syndrome (p. 180)

3A12

Histiocytosis X (Hand-Schüller-Christian's disease) (p. 143)

3B13

Blood dyscrasia: acute monocytic leukemia (p. 149)

3B14

Wegener's granulomatosis (p. 212)

3B15

Fibrous gingival hyperplasia caused by diphenylhydantoin sodium (p. 112)

3B16

Buccal exostoses and inflammatory gingival hyperplasia (pp. 87, 122)

3B17

Primary herpetic gingivostomatitis (p. 141)

3B18

Recurrent necrotizing ulcerative gingivostomatitis (p. 167)

3B19

Pemphigus vulgaris (p. 182)

3B20

Chronic periodontitis (p. 133)

3B21 and 3B22

Advanced chronic periodontitis (p. 133)

3B23

Pericoronitis (p. 186)

3B24

Malignant primary neoplasm: squamous cell carcinoma (p. 198)

3C25

Squamous cell carcinoma (p. 198)

3C26

Papilloma (p. 180)

3C27

Malignant neoplasm: fibrosarcoma (p. 119)

3C28

Inflammatory fibrous hyperplasia (denture injury tumor, epulis fissuratum) (p. 110)

3C29

Pyogenic granuloma (p. 191)

3C30

Fibrous gingival hyperplasia: with secondary ulceration (p. 122)

3C31
Pyogenic granuloma (p. 191)

3C32
Peripheral giant cell granuloma (p. 130)

3C33
Pyogenic granuloma. Consideration: Hypoprothrombinemia due to liver disease because the patient had obstructive jaundice (p. 191)

3C34
Tori mandibularis (p. 206)

3C35
Amalgam tattoo (p. 69)

3C36
Lentigo maligna melanoma (p. 148)

3D37
Exogenous pigmentation: silver pigmentation (p. 197)

3D38
Blood dyscrasia: thrombocytopenic purpura (p. 204)

3D39
Hematoma: secondary to vomiting (p. 138)

3D40
Hematoma (p. 138)

3D41
Infectious mononucleosis (p. 148)

3D42
Herpangina (p. 140)

3D43, 3D44, and 3D45
Benign mucous membrane pemphigoid (p. 84)

3D46
Inflammatory papillary hyperplasia (palatal papillomatosis) (p. 179)

3D47
Denture sore mouth (denture stomatitis) (p. 110)

3D48
Atrophic candidiasis (p. 110)

3E49
Nicotinic stomatitis (p. 169)

3E50
Leukoplakia: moderate epithelial dysplasia (p. 145)

3E51
Squamous cell carcinoma (p. 198)

3E52
Malignant lymphoma: lymphosarcoma (p. 157)

3E53
Salivary gland neoplasm: pleomorphic adenoma (p. 188)

3E54
Dentoalveolar abscess (p. 184)

3E55
"Fibroma" (p. 122)

3E56
Torus palatinus (p. 207)

3E57
Submucous cleft palate (p. 99)

3E58
Cleft palate associated with Apert's syndrome (p. 79)

3E59
Bifid uvula (p. 85)

3E60
Tertiary syphilis (gumma) (p. 201)

CHAPTER 4

Teeth

Before you read the patient histories, consult the preface for directions on how to use this atlas.

Patient Histories

4A1

This third molar tooth was extracted from a 23-year-old woman.

4A2

A 26-year-old man presented at the emergency clinic with pain in his upper central incisor. He had received a blow to his face while playing baseball.

4A3

This 11-year-old male adolescent was brought to the clinic for evaluation by his mother, who had a similar dental appearance.

4A4

A 12-year-old male adolescent had this dental appearance. No member of his immediate family was similarly affected.

4A5 and 4A6

A 6-year-old boy had this dentition. The patient had very thin and scanty scalp hair, dry skin, and absence of eyelashes. A composite radiograph is also shown. The patient was said to look identical to his maternal grandfather.

4A7 and 4A8

An 8-year-old boy was brought to the clinic by his parents because his newly erupted anterior teeth had a strange shape.

4A9

This 24-year-old man recalled having had infection on the anterior maxilla associated with one of his primary incisors.

4A10
A 31-year-old man had this dental appearance. He relates no history of trauma or periapical inflammation during the time of permanent crown formation.

4A11 and 4A12
A 32-year-old female technician from Taiwan complained of pain and swelling in the left mandibular area of 3 days' duration.

4B13
This condition was found in a 28-year-old woman during radiographic examination.

4B14
This 64-year-old woman, a refugee from South Vietnam, presented with this dental appearance.

4B15
A 40-year-old woman presented herself for "capping" of the anterior teeth. The patient had a hiatus hernia.

4B16 and 4B17
A 7-year-old girl had these dental findings. Her father and a sister had similar dentitions. A radiograph of her sister's anterior mandibular teeth is also shown.

4B18 and 4B19
This 21-year-old woman, a candy maker by occupation, came to the dental school to "have her teeth fixed." She had not had regular dental examinations and usually went only for extractions. The upper left central incisor had caused some pain 3 weeks previously.

4B20
An 8-year-old boy with these dental findings had no history of medications during the time of tooth formation. The child lived in a city where the fluoride content of the water was controlled. The child was otherwise healthy.

4B21
A 32-year-old woman complained about the appearance of her teeth. As a child she had lived in a rural area and her family had had their own water supply.

4B22
This 5-year-old boy presented this tooth discoloration. The mother stated that he had been a "yellow child" at birth and had needed a blood transfusion. The child had never had any antibiotic therapy. The family history was unremarkable.

4B23

A 14-year-old male adolescent, on routine dental examination, was found to have this dental appearance. A younger brother and the patient's mother had similar dental findings. There was no history of medication during pregnancy.

4B24 and 4C25

A 12-year-old male adolescent had this dental appearance. According to his mother, the patient had had a severe otitis media in infancy. This was treated with some sort of antibiotic. The next frame shows the same patient under an ultraviolet lamp.

4C26

A 25-year-old woman had this dentition. A sister of the patient's father had similar dental findings. The patient thought her father might have the same condition but to a lesser degree.

4C27

A 9-year-old boy with this dental appearance had a family history of similar tooth abnormalities.

4C28

This is the appearance of a 15-year-old male patient following removal of orthodontic bands and appliances.

4C29

This 5-year-old girl was brought to the clinic by her mother.

4C30

A 14-year-old male adolescent complained of not being able to keep his teeth white.

4C31

A 56-year-old woman complained of a burning sensation in her mouth, lips, and eyes. She also had a history of pain in the joints.

4C32

This 81-year-old woman was a conscientious tooth brusher and presented herself for routine examination.

4C33

A 35-year-old man had diffuse dental pain. The patient had never visited a dentist in his life.

4C34

A 30-year-old woman had these radiographic dental findings. Her teeth had an opalescent, bluish color and they cracked very easily. The patient's father and a brother had the same findings.

4C35

A 45-year-old woman presented herself for routine radiographic examination.

4C36

These radiographs correspond to two brothers aged 30 and 35 years who had teeth that readily exfoliated. Their mother had lost all of her teeth in a similar way.

4D37

This is a routine pantograph of a 9-year-old boy.

4D38

This condition was observed in a 9-year-old girl.

4D39

This is a radiograph of an 18-year-old female adolescent with missing anterior teeth.

4D40

This is a radiograph of a 16-year-old female adolescent. She had been hit by a truck and dragged for several yards when she was 4 years old. A week after hospital discharge the patient became aware of a swelling in the left maxillary cuspid area.

4D41

A 28-year-old woman complained of severe pain associated with her upper lateral and cuspid teeth.

4D42 and 4D43

A 25-year-old woman had had her last dental treatment 6 years ago, when silicate restorations were placed in her maxillary incisor teeth. This asymptomatic lateral incisor is now nonvital.

4D44 and 4D45

A 30-year-old man returned from a 6-month tour of military duty in Vietnam. Owing to climatic conditions he had consumed approximately thirty 16-ounce bottles of a commercial cola daily but decreased his consumption when he returned to a temperate climate. The black lesions were leathery on probing.

4D46

A 63-year-old man had had a lymphoma affecting the cervical lymph nodes 3 years previously for which he received radiation therapy. He now complained of a dry mouth and a burning sensation of the tongue. On clinical examination the tongue was found to have obvious candidiasis.

4D47 and 4D48

A 39-year-old woman came to the dental school for routine care of her teeth. The maxillary lateral incisor was noncarious but responded negatively to vitality tests. The patient recollected that the tooth had been sore after a fall on the ice a year ago.

4E49

A 15-year-old male adolescent had extensive active caries. This asymptomatic lesion, present for 8 months, had grown slowly.

4E50 and 4E51

This 6-year-old female Vietnamese refugee was accompanied by her older brother. He related an episode of swelling and pain in the patient a week previously. The second primary molar was mobile and carious. There was a grayish slough in the affected area. A right submandibular lymph node was enlarged and tender.

4E52

A 25-year-old man complained of constant severe boring pain at an extraction site 2 days after surgery. The extraction procedure was difficult. Gel foam and a suture had been placed upon completion.

4E53 and 4D54

A 24-year-old female was found to have this gingival lesion. A roentgenogram is shown in the next frame. The patient had no symptoms.

4E55

This is a radiograph of a 46-year-old woman complaining of pain associated with her first molar. Results of vitality tests were equivocal.

4E56

This 19-year-old male adolescent complained of marked pain in his second molar of a few days' duration.

4E57

This is a radiograph from a 37-year-old man. The patient complained of long-standing pain in the area.

4E58 and 4E59

A 35-year-old woman regularly attended a dental school for treatment. One year previously, a Class V gold foil restoration had been placed in the mandibular second premolar as an examination test case. Eight months previously a similar restoration had been placed in the first premolar. She complained of a painful swelling of her face, the two premolars being tender to touch and mobile. Her temperature was 101°F.

4E60

This roentgenogram is from an 8-year-old boy who complained of marked enlargement in the bicuspid area. According to his parents the growth had developed slowly over the last 2 months. There was slight pain on palpation. The patient was otherwise healthy.

Differential Diagnoses

4A1
Enamel pearl (enameloma, enamel drop)
Gemination

4A2
Abrasion
Fractured tooth
Peg-shaped tooth

4A3
Supernumerary tooth (mesiodens)

4A4
Congenital syphilis (Hutchinson's incisors)
Conoid central incisors

4A5 and 4A6
Hypohidrotic ectodermal dysplasia
Incontinentia pigmenti
Other forms of ectodermal dysplasia

4A7 and 4A8
Concrescence
Fusion
Gemination
Mesiodens
Supernumerary teeth

4A9
Amelogenesis imperfecta
Enamel hypoplasia (Turner's tooth)
Trauma

4A10
Attrition
Congenital syphilis (mulberry molar)
Enamel hypoplasia

4A11 and 4A12
Dentinogenesis imperfecta
Periapical abscess (acute)
Retained primary tooth

4B13
Dens in dente
External resorption
Internal resorption

4B14
Abrasion
Attrition
Enamel hypoplasia
Exogenous stain

4B15
Abrasion
Attrition
Bruxism
Erosion

4B16 and 4B17
Amelogenesis imperfecta
Dentinogenesis imperfecta
Erosion

4B18 and 4B19

Active occupational dental caries
Chronic marginal gingivitis
Dental sinus
Periapical granuloma

4B20

Enamel hypoplasia (Turner's tooth)
Exogenous pigmentation
Fluorosis
Marginal gingivitis

4B21

Amelogenesis imperfecta
Fluorosis
Rampant caries

4B22

Hereditary opalescent dentin
  (dentinogenesis imperfecta)
Pigmentation due to Rh
  incompatibility (erythroblastosis
  foetalis)
Tetracycline stain

4B23

Amelogenesis imperfecta
Dentinogenesis and osteogenesis
  imperfecta
Hereditary opalescent dentin
  (dentinogenesis imperfecta)

4B24 and 4C25

Amelogenesis imperfecta
Fluorosis
Tetracycline-induced changes

4C26

Amelogenesis imperfecta
Caries
Fluorosis

4C27

Amelogenesis imperfecta
Fluorosis

4C28

Caries
Chronic gingivitis
Enamel hypocalcification
Enamel hypoplasia

4C29

Black stain
Calculus
Caries

4C30

Calculus
Caries
Erythroblastosis foetalis
Green stain
Physiologic melanotic pigmentation
  of gingiva

4C31

Severe cervical caries secondary to diet
Severe cervical caries secondary to
  radiation therapy
Severe cervical caries secondary to
  Sjögren's syndrome

4C32

Abrasion
Attrition
Erosion
Periodontal disease

4C33

Dental caries
Multiple dental sinuses
Radiation caries

4C34

Amelogenesis imperfecta
Dentinal dysplasia (radicular type)
Dentinogenesis and osteogenesis
    imperfecta
Hereditary opalescent dentin
    (dentinogenesis imperfecta)

4C35

Dentinal dysplasia (radicular type)
Hereditary opalescent dentin
    (dentinogenesis imperfecta)
Pulp calcification (pulp stones)

4C36

Amelogenesis imperfecta
Dentinal dysplasia (radicular type)
Dentinogenesis and osteogenesis
    imperfecta
Hereditary opalescent dentin
    (dentinogenesis imperfecta)

4D37

Cynodontism
Dentinal dysplasia (radicular type)
Taurodontism

4D38

Dentinal dysplasia (radicular type)
Regional odontodysplasia (ghost
    teeth)
Resorption of unerupted teeth

4D39

Ankylosis
External resorption
Impacted tooth
Internal resorption

4D40

Dens in dente
Odontogenic neoplasm
Primordial cyst

4D41

Dens in dente
Periapical pathology

4D42 and 4D43

Globulomaxillary cyst
Necrotic tooth pulp
Odontogenic neoplasm
Periapical granuloma or cyst

4D44 and 4D45

Arrested dental caries secondary to
    soft drink consumption

4D46

Blood dyscrasia
Caries secondary to radiation
    xerostomia
Periodontal disease

4D47 and 4D48

Dental sinus
Physiologic melanotic pigmentation of
    gingiva
Pulp gangrene
Sclerosing osteitis
Traumatic necrosis of pulp

4E49

Chronic hyperplastic pulpitis
Peripheral giant cell granuloma
Pyogenic granuloma

4E50 and 4E51

Caries
Histiocytosis X
Juvenile periodontosis
Noma
Osteomyelitis
Periapical abscess

4E52

Dry socket
Neoplasia in tooth socket

4E53 and 4E54

Giant cell lesion
Gingival cyst
Lateral periodontal cyst
Odontogenic neoplasm

4E55

Lateral periodontal cyst
Odontogenic neoplasm
Periapical granuloma or radicular cyst
Residual cyst

4E56

Deep caries
Dentigerous cyst
Odontogenic keratocyst
Odontogenic neoplasm

4E57

Osteomyelitis
Periapical granuloma or radicular cyst

4E58 and 4E59

Acute cellulitis
Acute periapical abscess
Acute periodontitis
Traumatic pulp necrosis secondary to
    gold foil condensation

4E60

Bone neoplasm
Dentigerous cyst
Eruption cyst
Odontogenic neoplasm

Final Diagnoses

4A1

Enamel pearl (enameloma, enamel drop) (p. 114)

4A2

Fractured incisor tooth (p. 126)

4A3

Supernumerary tooth (mesiodens) (p. 161)

4A4

Conoid central incisors (p. 103)

4A5 and 4A6

Hypohidrotic ectodermal dysplasia (p. 146)

4A7 and 4A8

Gemination of central incisor with a supernumerary tooth (p. 129)

4A9

Enamel hypoplasia (Turner's tooth) (p. 113)

4A10

Congenital syphilis (mulberry molar) and enamel hypoplasia (p. 201)

4A11 and 4A12

Retained primary tooth with periapical abscess and no permanent successor (p. 184)

4B13

Internal resorption (p. 194)

4B14

Abrasion and exogenous stain due to chewing of betel nuts (pp. 67, 206)

4B15

Erosion: secondary to acid regurgitation (p. 115)

4B16 and 4B17

Amelogenesis imperfecta: smooth hypoplastic type (autosomal dominant) (p. 72)

4B18 and 4B19

Active occupational dental caries, chronic marginal gingivitis, dental sinus, and periapical granuloma (p. 90)

4B20

Enamel hypoplasia (Turner's tooth) and marginal gingivitis (p. 113)

4B21

Fluorosis: severe mottled enamel (p. 124)

4B22

Pigmentation due to Rh incompatibility (erythroblastosis foetalis) (p. 117)

4B23

Hereditary opalescent dentin (dentinogenesis imperfecta) (p. 139)

4B24 and 4C25

Tetracycline-induced changes: staining and enamel hypoplasia (p. 203)

4C26

Amelogenesis imperfecta: pitted hypoplastic type (autosomal dominant) (p. 72)

4C27

Amelogenesis imperfecta: snowcapped teeth (p. 72)

4C28

Caries following orthodontic banding and chronic gingivitis (p. 90)

4C29

Black stain (p. 206)

4C30

Green stain and physiologic melanotic pigmentation (pp. 160, 206)

4C31

Severe cervical caries secondary to Sjögren's syndrome (p. 92)

4C32

Abrasion: due to brushing (p. 67)

4C33

Dental caries and multiple dental sinuses (p. 90)

4C34

Hereditary opalescent dentin (dentinogenesis imperfecta) (p. 139)

4C35

Pulp calcification (pulp stones) (p. 190)

4C36

Dentinal dysplasia (radicular type) (p. 109)

4C37

Taurodontism. Consideration: Klinefelter's syndrome (because taurodontism in males can be associated with it) (p. 203)

4D38

Regional odontodysplasia (ghost teeth) (p. 170)

4D39

Impacted tooth with internal resorption (p. 194)

4D40

Dens in dente (p. 106)

4D41

Dens in dente with periapical pathology (p. 106)

4D42 and 4D43

Necrotic tooth pulp, secondary to unlined silicate restoration, and periapical granuloma or cyst (p. 189)

4D44 and 4D45

Arrested dental caries secondary to soft drink consumption (p. 90)

4D46

Caries secondary to radiation xerostomia (p. 91)

4D47 and 4D48

Dental sinus, physiologic melanotic pigmentation of gingiva, pulp gangrene, sclerosing osteitis, and traumatic necrosis of pulp (p. 107)

4E49

Chronic hyperplastic pulpitis (p. 191)

4E50 and 4E51

Caries with tissue loss secondary to a periapical abscess (p. 90)

4E52

Dry socket (p. 112)

4E53 and 4E54

Gingival cyst (p. 131)

4E55

Radicular cyst: associated with lateral canal from the mesial root of the molar tooth (p. 192

4E56

Odontogenic keratocyst, and deep caries in the second molar tooth (p. 171)

4E57

Periapical granuloma (p. 186)

4E58 and 4E59

Acute cellulitis, acute periapical abscess, acute periodontitis, and traumatic pulp necrosis secondary to gold foil condensation (p. 92)

4E60

Dentigerous cyst (p. 108)

CHAPTER 5

Bone

Before you read the patient histories, consult the preface for directions on how to use this atlas.

Patient Histories

5A1

A 32-year-old man had this intraoral appearance. These lumps had been present for many years; his father had similar findings.

5A2, 5A3, 5A4, and 5A5

A 62-year-old woman complained of a steady increase in the size of her maxilla. Her intraoral roentgenograms, her facial appearance, and her skull roentgenogram are also shown. The patient had had progressive hearing loss and lately had noticed some disturbance in her visual acuity. She also complained of pain in her legs on walking.

5A6

This roentgenogram is of a 42-year-old man who had had surgery for an adenocarcinoma of the large intestine. His mother had died at around age 40 of a malignant intestinal tumor. His sister has similar bony findings.

5A7 and 5A8

A 52-year-old woman presented with labial pigmentation and enlargement of the right maxilla and mandible of a year's duration. She complained of pain and recurring headaches. The oral radiographs are shown. A skeletal survey revealed a radiolucent lesion in the head of the right femur.

5A9 and 5A10

This 10-year-old girl was brought in because of the present facial and oral findings. Physical examination revealed some light-brown skin pigmentation over the chest. The patient's parents stated that this intraoral deformity had grown very slowly over the past 3 years. On surgical exposure the growth was found to be semisolid and was described as gritty to the knife.

5A11 and 5A12

This 18-year-old male complained of still having his deciduous teeth. Clinical examination revealed prominent frontal and parietal bones and a hypoplastic maxilla. A panoramic radiograph showed numerous unerupted teeth.

5B13 and 5B14

The facial appearance of this 12-year-old boy was similar to that of his mother. His pantographic radiograph is also shown. There were no other symptoms.

5B15 and 5B16

This 8-year-old boy presented with an intraoral growth of approximately 4 months' duration. The cortical plates were found to be extended, and slight pain was elicited on palpation. The patient was otherwise healthy. The corresponding pantographic radiograph is also shown.

5B17

This 25-year-old man complained of dull pain in the body of one side of the mandible. The teeth were vital. On radiographic examination this lesion was found. On surgical exposure the lesion was noted to be composed of solid soft tissue.

5B18

A 13-year-old female complained of a hard swelling of her left mandibular molar area. The corresponding teeth were vital. A radiograph revealed a well-defined radiolucency protruding between the roots of the molars. Aspiration of the lesion produced a straw-colored, clear fluid.

5B19

This 31-year-old woman complained of a unilateral dull ache in the body and ramus of her mandible. She had been seen by another dentist, who had extracted the second and third molars and curetted out a so-called cyst of the jaw. On surgical exposure the lesion was found to be composed of a soft tissue containing some empty spaces.

5B20

A 19-year-old man complained of unilateral anesthesia in his mandible. The lesion had been treated surgically 2 years previously with the diagnosis of "some sort of cyst." The patient was otherwise healthy. The second surgical exposure revealed a lesion comprising several cavities containing blood.

5B21

A 60-year-old man complained of a severe, unilateral, and persistent pain in the mandible. The teeth in the area were mobile. A radiologic skeletal survey demonstrated the presence of radiolucent lesions in the skull and the long bones.

5B22

This 58-year-old woman complained of pain near the mandibular premolars. According to the patient, the teeth had recently shifted position slightly. However, they were vital. The patient was otherwise healthy. On clinical examination a yellowish, cheesy material was exuded by pressure on this area.

5B23

A 26-year-old man complained of a unilateral, dull ache in the mandible. There was a history of previous extractions and mobility of teeth. On intraoral examination a marked cavitation of the alveolar ridge was observed. A skeletal bone survey was negative. Laboratory analyses were also noncontributory.

5B24

These roentgenograms are of a 48-year-old man with marked facial asymmetry of 6 months' duration following a traumatic incident. There was no other symptomatology. A skeletal survey was negative.

5C25

An 8-year-old boy had slight facial deformity and these radiologic findings. The patient had been treated elsewhere and no final diagnosis had been established. The patient had slight paresthesia on this side.

5C26

A 63-year-old woman related a 40-year history of a painless, bilateral, slow-growing enlargement of her mandible that had stopped expanding 10 years previously. The patient had since had chronic osteomyelitis.

5C27

These findings were discovered upon routine radiologic survey of a 55-year-old woman. The patient had no symptoms.

5C28

A 28-year-old man on routine intraoral examination was found to have the present radiologic appearance with no symptoms.

5C29

The present findings were discovered on routine radiologic survey of a 32-year-old man. The patient had no symptoms.

5C30

A 25-year-old woman sought consultation for mild pain from a restored first mandibular molar. A periapical radiograph revealed an ill-defined radiopacity surrounding the apex of both roots.

5C31

An 18-year-old woman had had this slow-growing sessile bony enlargement of the mandibular premolar area for the past 6 years. The adjacent teeth were vital.

5C32

A 19-year-old man complained of mobility of his mandibular anterior teeth as well as a dull, persistent bone pain. There was slight facial asymmetry in the area that had developed rapidly over the last month.

5C33

A 56-year-old woman complained of persistent pain and tooth mobility in the mandibular bicuspid-molar area. The patient related a history of a "tumor" removed from her breast a few years previously.

5C34 and 5C35

A 64-year-old man complained of a persistent pain in his mandible. The patient also related symptoms of tiredness and dizziness. The intraoral roentgenogram is shown followed by the skull roentgenogram of the same patient.

5C36

Skull roentgenograms of this 5½-year-old girl were taken because the patient complained of tooth mobility and presented clinically with exophthalmos. A roentgenologic bone survey was done and similar lesions were observed in the long bones.

5D37

This intraoral roentgenogram is from a 45-year-old man who complained of tooth mobility and severe pain in the mandibular premolar area. A fungating, easily bleeding mass was observed intraorally. The patient was otherwise in apparent good health.

5D38

A 41-year-old man had this intraosseous lesion, discovered on routine radiographic examination. There was no evidence of cortical expansion, crepitation, or other symptoms referable to the lesion. The patient had been on diphenylhydantoin therapy for many years. The teeth in the area were vital.

5D39

This roentgenogram is from a 50-year-old woman whose present findings were discovered on routine radiographic examination. The patient was without symptoms.

5D40

A 28-year-old woman was found to have a recurrent radiolucency that had grown to this size 10 years after it had first been curetted. The adjacent teeth were vital.

5D41

This 9-year-old boy complained of persistent pain in the anterior mandible. Clinically, displacement and mobility of teeth were noted. A firm, hard swelling that had developed over the last month was present on the chin.

5D42

This intraoral roentgenogram was obtained during routine dental examination of a 26-year-old man. According to the referring dentist, these teeth were vital. Repeated vitality tests yielded equivocal results. The incisal edges of the mandibular incisors had marked wear facets.

5D43

These findings were observed in the routine radiologic examination of a 35-year-old woman. The patient had no symptoms. Roentgenograms taken 10 years prior to the present consultation demonstrated areas of radiolucency where the present alterations are observed.

5D44

These radiopacities were noted during routine examination of a 24-year-old man. They were asymptomatic, and the patient was in good health.

5D45

This intraoral roentgenogram was obtained from a 25-year-old woman. No clinical symptomatology was associated with this finding.

5D46

A 24-year-old man complained of a unilateral, dull, intermittent pain in the body of his mandible that was alleviated by aspirin. The symptoms had been present for about 3 months. On palpation a small nodule was noted in the area. The adjacent teeth were vital.

5D47

This roentgenogram was obtained from a 63-year-old man who complained of acute unilateral, persistent pain in the body of his mandible. Clinical examination revealed a purulent exudate containing some bony debris. There was a history of a fall that had occurred 2 months prior to consultation.

5D48 and 5E49

This 21-year-old man had struck his chin on the steering wheel of an automobile in an accident 4 months before consultation. The mandibular incisors were nonvital. A radiograph of the area is also presented.

5E50 and 5E51

A 6-month-old girl had these ocular findings. An X ray of her lower extremities also is shown. The child was born with several intrauterine fractures. The patient's mother had a history of easily fractured bones, and her teeth were yellowish in color with enamel that flaked off very easily.

5E52

This radiograph of a 21-year-old woman shows an apparent mandibular deformity. The patient was without symptoms. The lesion had developed slowly over the past 5 years.

5E53

A 7-year-old boy complained of a hard swelling on the left side of his mandible and of pain from decayed primary molars. An intraoral radiograph revealed periapical pathology in both deciduous molars. An occlusal X ray taken after extraction of the offending teeth demonstrated a bony enlargement.

5E54

This 30-year-old woman, in apparent good health, had a 4-month history of progressive enlargement of the maxillary tuberosity. There was some crepitation on palpation and the patient experienced slight pain.

5E55

This is a routine dental radiograph from a 50-year-old man.

5E56

This radiograph of a 17-year-old female was taken because the patient was complaining of progressive enlargement of the area. The lesion was hard on palpation and the patient was otherwise asymptomatic.

5E57

This 12-year-old female had a slight enlargement of the maxillary canine-premolar area. There was no pain or other symptomatology. The patient was otherwise in good health.

5E58

A 21-year-old man complained of progressive displacement of the maxillary lateral and canine teeth. Clinically, there was slight enlargement of the area, and on palpation this region was found to be crepitant.

5E59

A 55-year-old man complained of persistent deep bone pain in this area with mobility of teeth. The patient was pale and had lost 20 pounds in the last 2 months.

5E60

This 62-year-old man complained of soreness beneath his denture in the area of the incisive papilla. The radiograph is shown.

Differential Diagnoses

5A1

Buccal exostoses
Chondromas
Osteomas

5A2, 5A3, 5A4, and 5A5

Fibrous dysplasia of bone
Multiple myeloma
Osteitis deformans (Paget's disease of bone)

5A6

Diffuse sclerosing osteomyelitis
Osteomatosis (intestinal polyposis syndrome, Gardner's syndrome)
Osteopetrosis
Polyostotic fibrous dysplasia

5A7 and 5A8

Hyperparathyroidism
Osteitis deformans (Paget's disease of bone)
Polyostotic fibrous dysplasia

5A9 and 5A10

Benign bone neoplasm
Monostotic fibrous dysplasia
Neurofibromatosis of von Recklinghausen
Odontogenic neoplasm

5A11 and 5A12

Cleidocranial dysplasia (cleidocranial dysostosis)
Pyknodysostosis

5B13 and 5B14

Cherubism
Multiple odontogenic keratocysts
Polyostotic fibrous dysplasia

5B15 and 5B16

Bone neoplasia
Central giant cell granuloma
Monostotic fibrous dysplasia
Odontogenic cyst
Odontogenic neoplasm

5B17

Bone neoplasm
Odontogenic cyst
Odontogenic neoplasm
Traumatic bone cyst

5B18

Aneurysmal bone cyst
Odontogenic cyst
Periapical cyst and/or granuloma secondary to caries
Traumatic bone cyst

5B19

Bone neoplasm
Neurogenic neoplasm
Odontogenic keratocyst
Odontogenic neoplasm
Residual cyst

5B20

Aneurysmal bone cyst
Bone neoplasm
Central hemangioma
Monostotic fibrous dysplasia
Odontogenic neoplasm

5B21

Histiocytosis X
  (Hand-Schüller-Christian's disease)
Metastatic neoplasm
Multiple myeloma

5B22

Bone neoplasm
Odontogenic cyst
Odontogenic neoplasm
Osteomyelitis

5B23

Bone neoplasm
Developmental lingual mandibular
  salivary gland depression
Histiocytosis X: eosinophilic
  granuloma of bone
Odontogenic cyst
Odontogenic neoplasm

5B24

Bone neoplasm
Monostotic fibrous dysplasia
Odontogenic neoplasm
Osteitis deformans (Paget's disease of
  bone)

5C25

Bone neoplasm
Monostotic fibrous dysplasia
Odontogenic neoplasm
Sclerosing osteitis

5C26

Bone neoplasm
Chronic osteomyelitis
Florid osseous dysplasia
Osteitis deformans (Paget's disease of
  bone)

5C27

Bone neoplasm
Chronic focal sclerosing osteitis
  (condensing osteitis)
Odontogenic neoplasm

5C28

Cementoblastoma
Gigantiform cementoma
Hypercementosis
Osteoblastoma
Sclerosing osteitis
  (condensing osteitis)

5C29

Cementifying fibroma
Gigantiform cementoma
Hypercementosis
Sclerosing osteitis
  (condensing osteitis)

5C30

Chronic periodontitis
Gigantiform cementoma
Hypercementosis
Sclerosing osteitis
  (condensing osteitis)

5C31

Bone neoplasm
Metastatic neoplasm
Monostotic fibrous dysplasia
Odontogenic neoplasm

5C32

Bone neoplasm
Periodontosis
Soft tissue neoplasm

5C33

Bone neoplasm
Metastatic neoplasm
Odontogenic keratocyst
Osteomyelitis

5C34 and 5C35

Bone neoplasm
Histiocytosis X
(Hand-Schüller-Christian's disease)
Metastatic neoplasm
Multiple myeloma
Osteitis deformans (Paget's disease of
bone)

5C36

Bone neoplasm
Chloromas associated with leukemia
Histiocytosis X
(Hand-Schüller-Christian's disease)
Metastatic neoplasm

5D37

Bone neoplasm
Metastatic neoplasm
Odontogenic neoplasm
Periodontitis
Squamous cell carcinoma

5D38

Aneurysmal bone cyst
Focal bone marrow defect
Odontogenic neoplasm
Traumatic bone cyst

5D39

Bone neoplasm
Mental foramen
Neurogenic neoplasm
Odontogenic cyst

5D40

Giant cell granuloma
Odontogenic cyst
Odontogenic neoplasm
Periapical cyst or granuloma
Traumatic bone cyst

5D41

Bone neoplasm

Monostotic fibrous dysplasia
Odontogenic neoplasm

5D42

Bone neoplasm
Cementoma
Periapical cemental dysplasia
Periapical granuloma or cyst

5D43

Cementoma
Chronic periodontitis
Florid osseous dysplasia
Gigantiform cementoma
Periapical cemental dysplasia
Sclerosing osteitis (condensing osteitis)

5D44

Foreign bodies
Multiple osteomas
Tori mandibularis
X-ray artifact

5D45

Foreign body
Impacted supernumerary tooth
Odontogenic neoplasm

5D46

Bone neoplasm
Monostotic fibrous dysplasia
Garré's osteitis (chronic osteomyelitis
with proliferative periostitis)

5D47

Bone neoplasm
Fractured jaw
Hyperparathyroidism
Multiple myeloma
Osteomyelitis

5D48 and 5E49

External resorption
Facial scar
Horizontal alveolar bone fracture
Traumatic necrosis of tooth pulps

5E50 and 5E51

Achondroplasia
Dentinogenesis imperfecta
Osteogenesis imperfecta

5E52

Aneurysmal bone cyst
Benign bone neoplasm
Central giant cell granuloma
Monostotic fibrous dysplasia
Odontogenic neoplasm

5E53

Bone neoplasm
Garré's osteitis (chronic osteomyelitis
    with proliferative periosteitis)
Odontogenic neoplasm
Subperiosteal abscess

5E54

Bone neoplasm
Monostotic fibrous dysplasia
Neoplasm of maxillary sinus
Odontogenic neoplasm
Salivary gland neoplasm

5E55

Bone neoplasm
Metastatic neoplasm
Neoplasm of maxillary sinus
Odontogenic neoplasm

5E56

Bone neoplasm
Monostotic fibrous dysplasia
Odontogenic neoplasm

5E57

Bone neoplasm
Odontogenic neoplasm

5E58

Bone neoplasm
Globulomaxillary cyst
Odontogenic cyst
Odontogenic neoplasm

5E59

Blood dyscrasia
Bone neoplasm
Malignant lymphoma
Odontogenic neoplasm

5E60

Enlarged incisive canal
Nasopalatine cyst
Residual cyst

Final Diagnoses

5A1

Buccal exostoses (p. 87)

5A2, 5A3, 5A4, and 5A5

Osteitis deformans (Paget's disease of bone) (p. 178)

5A6

Osteomatosis (intestinal polyposis syndrome, Gardner's syndrome) (p. 127)

5A7 and 5A8

Polyostotic fibrous dysplasia (p. 121)

5A9 and 5A10

Monostotic fibrous dysplasia (p. 119)

5A11 and 5A12

Cleidocranial dysplasia (cleidocranial dysostosis) (p. 102)

5B13 and 5B14

Cherubism (p. 97)

5B15 and 5B16

Odontogenic neoplasm: ameloblastic fibroma (p. 70)

5B17

Bone neoplasm: ossifying fibroma (p. 173)

5B18

Traumatic bone cyst (p. 208)

5B19

Odontogenic neoplasm: ameloblastoma (p. 71)

5B20

Aneurysmal bone cyst (p. 77)

5B21

Multiple myeloma (p. 165)

5B22

Odontogenic keratocyst: with squamous cell carcinoma (p. 171)

5B23

Histiocytosis X: Eosinophilic granuloma of bone (p. 143)

5B24

Odontogenic neoplasm: calcifying epithelial odontogenic tumor (Pindborg's tumor) (p. 86)

5C25

Odontogenic neoplasm: complex odontoma (p. 172)

5C26

Florid osseous dysplasia (p. 123)

5C27

Chronic focal sclerosing osteitis (condensing osteitis) (p. 195)

5C28

Sclerosing osteitis (condensing osteitis) (p. 195)

5C29

Hypercementosis (p. 144)

5C30

Sclerosing osteitis (condensing osteitis) (p. 195)

5C31

Monostotic fibrous dysplasia (p. 119)

5C32

Bone neoplasm: osteosarcoma (p. 176)

5C33

Metastatic neoplasm: adenocarcinoma from breast (p. 161)

5C34 and 5C35

Multiple myeloma (p. 165)

5C36

Histiocytosis X
(Hand-Schüller-Christian's disease)
(p. 143)

5D37

Metastatic neoplasm: renal carcinoma
(p. 161)

5D38

Odontogenic neoplasm: myxofibroma
(p. 172)

5D39

Odontogenic cyst: residual cyst
(p. 192)

5D40

Odontogenic cyst: odontogenic
keratocyst (p. 171)

5D41

Bone neoplasm: osteosarcoma (p. 176)

5D42

Periapical granuloma (p. 186)

5D43

Chronic periodontitis and periapical
cemental dysplasia (pp. 133, 185)

5D44

Tori mandibularis (p. 206)

5D45

Odontogenic neoplasm: compound
odontoma (p. 172)

5D46

Bone neoplasm: osteoid osteoma
(p. 175)

5D47

Fractured jaw: with osteomyelitis
(pp. 126, 175)

5D48 and 5E49

External resorption, facial scar,
horizontal alveolar bone fracture, and
traumatic necrosis of tooth pulps
(p. 194)

5E50 and 5E51

Osteogenesis imperfecta (p. 174)

5E52

Central giant cell granuloma (p. 129)

5E53

Garré's osteitis (chronic osteomyelitis
with proliferative periosteitis) (p. 128)

5E54

Odontogenic neoplasm: myxoma
(p. 172)

5E55

Odontogenic neoplasm:
ameloblastoma (p. 71)

5E56

Odontogenic neoplasm: complex
odontoma (p. 172)

5E57

Odontogenic neoplasm: adenomatoid
odontogenic tumor (p. 69)

5E58

Globulomaxillary cyst (p. 134)

5E59

Malignant lymphoma: histiocytic type
(reticulum cell sarcoma, malignant
histiocytoma) (p. 157)

5E60

Nasopalatine cyst (p. 166)

PART 2 SHORT DESCRIPTIONS OF ORAL DISEASES

Short Descriptions of Oral Diseases

Abrasion (4B14; 4C32)

Abrasion is the pathologic wearing off of calcified dental tissue that generally occurs as a result of a traumatic process.

Clinical Features

Abrasion can occur on any tooth surface. The most frequently affected area is the gingival one-third of the buccal surface of the crown, where it is most likely a consequence of improper horizontal toothbrushing, especially with an abrasive toothpaste. In this particular location it will manifest itself as a saucerlike cavitation at the same level in several teeth. This type of lesion routinely extends into the cementum with consequent gingival recession. The bottom of this cavity is well polished, and in extreme cases the pulp can be seen by transparency. Other types of abrasion can be observed at either the incisal edge or the occlusal surfaces, generally in patients with closed bite or with teeth-antagonizing prostheses. Individuals such as carpenters or seamstresses may have a notch at the incisal edge of the tooth or teeth with which they hold nails or pins. Some pipe smokers also may present a notch in the teeth with which the pipe stem is held. Whatever the etiologic agent, abrasion is manifested as a loss of enamel and dentin. The cause of this loss is easily ascertained by questioning the patient.

Differential Diagnosis (see pp. 47, 48)

The differential diagnosis should include attrition, erosion (4B15), and cervical caries (4C31).

Laboratory Aids

None.

Treatment

Gingival restorations and occlusal splints are employed in restoring aesthetic appearance and vertical dimension.

Actinomycosis (1D46)

Actinomycosis is a chronic granulomatous and suppurative infection caused by bacteria of the genus *Actinomyces*. These bacteria grow in a manner similar to that of fungi, that is, with branching filaments. Actinomycosis is produced in humans chiefly by two varieties of the bacteria—the so-called *Actinomyces israelii* and *Actinomyces odontolyticus*. Other microorganisms are also known to produce this disease in humans. *Actinomyces bovis* produces the disease in animals.

Clinical Features

Cervical actinomycosis initially can be considered a subacute process generally preceded by a history of recent dental extraction. Occasionally, it may complicate a fracture that has been exposed to the oral cavity. The microorganism is thought to be a commensal in the oral cavity. The condition is slightly painful and is characterized by an area of enlargement due to progressive swelling, most likely occurring in the mandible. The bacteria grow, forming intrabony granulomas that eventually create a sinus tract. When the condition occurs in the mandible, the sinus frequently drains at the level of the angle. The affected skin becomes purple in color, and the granuloma has a woody consistency. The purulent discharge contains the typical sulfur granules. If the lesion is not treated, trismus and multiple-draining sinus may develop. Complications can occur in the form of osteomyelitis of the affected bone. Extension of the process into the orbit or even the base of the skull is known to occur. The disease is chronic, and the patient may occasionally present with a slightly increased body temperature.

Differential Diagnosis (see p. 11)

All of the granulomatous diseases (1D43) as well as abscess of dental origin (1D42; 4E58) should be included in the differential diagnosis, but the identification of the multiple sinus and the sulfur granules should lead to a positive diagnosis for actinomycosis.

Laboratory Aids

The causative agent can be very easily identified, either by culture or by direct examination of the exudate, which will reveal the sulfur granules. Microscopically, the colonies will present hyphae, which are very typical for this condition. Sedimentation rate will be elevated and the white blood cell count might reveal a mild anemia.

Treatment

The condition is treated with appropriate doses of antibiotics.

Adenomatoid Odontogenic Tumor (5E57)

Adenomatoid odontogenic tumor is a benign neoplasm generally associated with the crown of an unerupted tooth. Some authors consider this entity a hamartoma.

Clinical Features

The condition presents as a slow-growing, painless enlargement—generally of the anterior maxilla but occasionally of the anterior mandible—overlying or replacing an unerupted tooth. The lesion may occupy a portion of the wall of a dentigerous cyst, though it generally has a lateral distribution to the crown and tooth root. It presents as a predominantly radiolucent lesion with a thin, radiopaque margin, and it may contain varying amounts of radiopaque flecks. The patients are most commonly females in their second decade. The behavior of the lesion is characterized by an extremely benign, slow growth with encapsulation. The only complication arises from displacement of the adjacent teeth.

Differential Diagnosis (see p. 62)

The presence of fleck calcification in radiographs is quite indicative. Nevertheless, in older individuals Pindborg's tumor should be considered in the differential diagnosis.

Laboratory Aids

It is extremely important that this lesion be differentiated from the ameloblastoma. Microscopically, glandlike structures give the tumor its name, and focal calcifications can contribute to the radiographic appearance of the tumor.

Treatment

Surgical enucleation and, if necessary, orthodontic restoration is the indicated treatment. The lesion does not return after removal.

Amalgam Tattoo (3C35)

Amalgam tattoo is a pigmentation of the oral mucosa caused by entrapment of dental amalgam fragments in soft tissue.

Clinical Features

This pigmentation is a common, irregular, blue-black macule of variable size found in any area of the oral mucosa where the silver compounds of amalgam may accidentally have fallen into small wounds or abrasions during cutting of a tooth, packing of a restoration, or extraction of a tooth containing a restoration. The metallic fragments can be detected radiographically. The pigmentation is inert and has no complications.

Differential Diagnosis (see p. 37)

Melanin-producing lesions, such as nevus, melanoma, ephelis (1C28), and lentigo maligna melanoma (3C36) should be considered. Physiologic melanin deposition is seen in blacks, orientals, and whites in varying degrees according to racial extraction (4C30; 4D47). Intraorally, this is generally confined to the attached gingiva and follows the normal wavy gingival contour. Variation in color depends on the amount of pigment deposited in the epithelium. Rarely, physiologic pigmentation is seen in other areas of the oral mucosa.

Several heavy metals—notably mercury, lead, and bismuth—produce gingival pigmentation, but the pigmentation is confined to the marginal gingiva. The color varies from blue to black and has a linear distribution along the gingival sulcus. Mercury poisoning also produces oral ulcerations, hemorrhage, and sialorrhea. Silver pigmentation from silver-containing medications gives a diffuse metallic blue discoloration seen mostly in the exposed area of the skin but also intraorally. Patients who have used nasal drops containing silver may have palatal pigmentation (3D37). Antimalarial drugs such as chloroquine also will produce intraoral pigmentation.

Laboratory Aids

A variety of histochemical stains can discriminate among exogenous and endogenous pigments.

Treatment

None.

Ameloblastic Fibroma (5B15 and 5B16)

The ameloblastic fibroma is an odontogenic neoplasm that is considered a true mixed tumor. In this neoplasm, both epithelial and connective tissue components proliferate, but they never produce calcified tissues.

Clinical Features

Eighty percent of these neoplasms develop in the mandibular molar region. The majority of the cases occur in young children. The average age of affected patients obtained from all reported cases of ameloblastic fibroma is 15 years. Both sexes are equally affected. Examples in older individuals have also been reported. Ameloblastic fibroma grows very slowly and generally does not present clinical symptomatology. Occasionally, a tumor may produce displacement of teeth and facial asymmetry. Radiographically it manifests as a unilocular (rarely multilocular), radiolucent lesion that generally has a very definite outline. The condition is entirely benign.

Differential Diagnosis (see p. 59)

The differential diagnosis should include a variety of lesions, such as other odontogenic tumors occurring in children, fibrous dysplasia, and central giant cell lesions (5E52). The condition differs from ameloblastoma in that it does not invade the neighboring tissues and has an entirely different histologic appearance.

Laboratory Aids

Biopsy will demonstrate a neoplastic proliferation of connective tissue that is very similar to the appearance of a developing tooth pulp. Within this embryonal connective tissue, islands of ameloblastic epithelium will be observed.

Treatment

The treatment is conservative surgery. Curettage will effect a positive cure.

Ameloblastoma (5B19; 5E55)

Ameloblastoma is an epithelial odontogenic neoplasm that is considered locally aggressive. It is thought to be derived from the dental lamina.

Clinical Features

These neoplasms occur equally in males and females with the average age at time of diagnosis being about 40 years. The tumor has been observed in individuals from ages 4 to 80 but is most frequently observed in the second or third decade. The mandible is affected in 80% of the cases, and the most frequent site of occurrence is the mandibular angle and the area of the third mandibular molar. When in the maxilla, it generally occurs in the area of the tuberosity. Some other sites also can be affected. The neoplasm grows very slowly and is essentially painless. It produces displacement of teeth in the area affected, as well as resorption of tooth roots. The tumor does not metastasize and is considered histologically benign but locally aggressive. The lesion can reach a considerable size and produce a large destruction of bone. When in the maxilla, it may invade the maxillary sinus and cause displacement of the orbit. Clinical examination demonstrates facial asymmetry in advanced cases. The tumor can also appear in the wall of a dentigerous cyst. Radiographically it presents a series of images, the most frequent one being described as a multilocular radiolucency with a soap bubble or honeycomb appearance. Unilocular varieties are also observed. Bone resorption and erosion of the cortical plate are evident. In advanced cases, erosion of the basilar portion of the mandible can also be observed, and secondary infection and secondary fractures might supervene.

Differential Diagnosis (see pp. 59, 62)

The differential diagnosis can include a great variety of lesions, including Pindborg's tumor (5B24), odontogenic myxoma (5E54), fibrous dysplasia, odontogenic keratocyst (4E56), and other neoplasms not necessarily odontogenic (including metastatic disease to the jaws).

Laboratory Aids

Biopsy will reveal the nature of the lesion.

Treatment

The treatment is surgical in all cases. Surgery should be performed in a hospital setting. The lesion should be eliminated with wide margins extending into normal tissues. In the maxilla, the surgical treatment needs to be much more aggressive because of the greater possibility for the tumor to spread into a more porous bone.

Amelogenesis Imperfecta
(4B16 and 4B17; 4C26 and 4C27)

Hereditary defects in enamel not associated with other systemic defects are known as amelogenesis imperfecta. Based upon clinical, histologic, and genetic criteria, amelogenesis imperfecta can be classified into hypoplastic, hypocalcified, and hypomaturation types.

Clinical Features

Hypoplastic types of amelogenesis imperfecta are those in which the enamel is thinner than normal. In enamel with normal thickness, subnormal hardness differentiates hypocalcified varieties from hypomaturation varieties. Hypomaturation amelogenesis imperfecta contains large amounts of enamel matrix that allow the tip of a dental explorer to penetrate under pressure, whereas hypocalcified enamel is of such a consistency that it can be easily scraped away. Table 1 illustrates the different nonsyndromal varieties of amelogenesis imperfecta.

Differential Diagnosis (see pp. 47, 48)

Dentinogenesis imperfecta and those severe cases of enamel hypoplasia produced by tetracycline should be considered. To distinguish among the different types of amelogenesis imperfecta, refer to Table 1.

Laboratory Aids

None.

TABLE 1. Classification of Amelogenesis Imperfecta

	Dentition Affected		Color of Enamel	Defect and Surface Affected	Miscellaneous
	Primary	Secondary			
Hypoplastic					
1. Pitted, autosomal dominant	+	+	Initially yellow-white, becomes pockmarked	Random pinpoint pits on labial and lingual	None
2. Local, autosomal dominant	+	+	Yellow-white to chalky white	Buccal middle one-third of enamel as horizontal row of pits or linear depression	None
3. Smooth, autosomal dominant	−	+	Yellow on eruption, later becomes opaque white to brownish	Thin, hard, glossy with smooth surface on buccal and lingual	Pulpal calcifications may be present in erupted and unerupted teeth. Multiple unerupted teeth undergoing resorption are common
4. Rough, autosomal dominant	+	+	Yellow-white on eruption	Thin, rough, hard on buccal and lingual	Impacted and partly resorbed teeth are rare but have been reported
5. Rough, autosomal recessive	+	+	Yellow, resembling dentin	Rough granular enamel on labial and lingual	Numerous teeth are missing in erupted dentition and are manifested radiographically as unerupted teeth undergoing resorption

SOURCE: Reprinted by permission of the publisher, from Sedano, Heddie O., Sauk, John Jr., and Gorlin, Robert J., *Oral Manifestations of Inherited Disorders*. Woburn: Butterworth Publishers, Inc., 1977.

TABLE 1 — *Continued*

	Dentition Affected		Color of Enamel	Defect and Surface Affected	Miscellaneous
	Primary	Secondary			
6. Smooth, X-linked dominant	+	+	Yellow-brown	Shiny thin occlusal and incisal abrasion	Females show vertical banding of hypoplastic and normal enamel consistent with Lyonization effect of genes on the X chromosome in heterozygous females. Anterior open bite is common
Hypomaturation					
1. Hypomaturation-hypoplastic with taurodontism, autosomal dominant	+	+	Shiny opaque white with irregular areas of yellow-brown mottling	Mottling and pitting of labial	This condition may be an incomplete expression of the tricho-dento-osseous syndrome
2. X-linked recessive	+	+	Primary teeth of males show opaque white. Permanent teeth show yellow-white color that stains with age. Females show alternating vertical bands of white opaque enamel	Translucent mottling in primary teeth of males on labial and lingual. Enamel in secondary dentition of males is normal thickness and may be penetrated with an explorer.	Females show vertical banding of hypomature and normal enamel consistent with Lyonization effect of genes on the X-chromosome in heterozygous females.

TABLE 1—*Continued*

| | Dentition Affected | | Color of Enamel | Defect and Surface Affected | Miscellaneous |
	Primary	Secondary			
3. Pigmented-autosomal recessive	+	+	Milky to shiny agar brown	Labial and lingual show normal thickness but hypomature enamel	Unerupted teeth may be present and undergo resorption
4. Snowcapped teeth	+	+	Opaque white	Hypomaturation of incisal or occlusal one-third	None
Hypocalcified					
1. Autosomal dominant	+	+	Newly erupted teeth are dull, lusterless, opaque white, honey colored or yellow-orange-brown	Labial and lingual are covered with cheesy, soft enamel	Anterior open bite and excessive calculus formation are common
2. Autosomal recessive	+	+	Same as dominant form	Same as dominant form	Clinically, radio-graphically, and histo-logically this recessive form is more severe than autosomal dominant hypocalcified amelogenesis imperfecta

Treatment

Ideally, the patient can be treated with full-mouth porcelain jackets and crown restorations.

Amyloidosis (2E56)

Amyloidosis is produced by the accumulation in tissues of an abnormal eosinophilic fibrillar material that is, in its major part, formed by cross-beta proteins similar to immunoglobulin light chains. Amyloidosis is classified as primary or secondary. Primary amyloidosis is seen associated with a large variety of chronic diseases, especially those associated with alterations in immunity and autoimmune reactions. Certain neoplasms, especially plasma cell dyscrasias, are associated with secondary amyloidosis. Among the most frequent chronic disorders presenting amyloidosis in later periods are tuberculosis, lupus erythematosus, rheumatoid arthritis, Hodgkin's disease, and multiple myeloma.

Clinical Features

Description will be confined to the primary form, which is the one that produces oral and perioral manifestations. Affected individuals show marked weakness, weight loss, neurologic manifestations, and, in the later periods, heart failure. The perioral skin, as well as areas of pressure, present ecchymoses and petechiae with a characteristic dark purple color. These lesions are known as amyloid tumors. In the primary form, amyloidosis is frequently deposited in the tongue, with consequent marked lingual enlargement, which interferes with normal mastication as well as speech. The tongue shows the imprint of all of the teeth in the dental arch. There is no pain associated with this tongue enlargement, but it may lead to dysphagia and obstruction of the air passages. Tongue mobility is consequently altered.

Differential Diagnosis (see p. 25)

Rarely could any other disorder be associated with macroglossia. The only exceptions are some inherited conditions that would be present from birth. Nevertheless, one should consider lymphedema as well as lymphangioma.

Laboratory Aids

Laboratory studies offer a great array of means helpful in diagnosis. Blood analyses will demonstrate anemia and leukocytosis. Sedimentation rate is generally elevated. Urine will show massive proteinurea. Electrophoresis will show low albumin and globulin levels. The most efficient means of diagnosis is biopsy. Tissue is easily obtained from the border of the tongue. Special stains with Congo red and other dyes will demonstrate the nature of the accumulated material, thus establishing the diagnosis.

Treatment

Treatment is entirely systemic and in the hands of the physician. Patients with primary amyloidosis generally have a very poor prognosis.

Aneurysmal Bone Cyst (5B20)

Aneurysmal bone cyst is a nonneoplastic lesion of bone generally consisting of several cavities filled with blood and deprived of an endothelial lining. Aneurysmal bone cyst is most common in the long bones and vertebrae, but it has also been reported in the clavicle and rib as well as in other bones. The etiology of aneurysmal bone cyst is probably a local circulatory disturbance causing an alteration in hemodynamics, with the formation of the cyst as a reactive lesion.

Clinical Features

Aneurysmal bone cyst constitutes about 1.5% of all nonodontogenic and nonepithelial cysts of the jaws. It is, therefore, a rare lesion in that location. A survey of aneurysmal bone cyst of the jaws (El Deeb, M., Sedano, H. O., and Waite, D., Aneurysmal bone cyst: Case presentation and review of the literature, *Int. J. Oral Surg.* 1980:9:301, indicates that 75% of the cases occurred in patients 20 years and younger, with a range in age of 6 to 59 years and a mean of 18 years. Fifty-five percent of the cases were found in the mandible and 45% in the maxilla. Females were affected in 53% of the cases; males, in the remaining 47%. The recurrence rate of the lesion is 25% for the jaw bones. The lesion occurs as a benign, localized, solitary swelling, the development of which may vary from a few weeks to several years. The growth is expansile in nature, and sometimes pain or paresthesia may accompany symptoms. Facial asymmetry is evident; intraorally displacement of teeth and erasure of sulci are also seen.

The radiographic features of aneurysmal bone cyst are not characteristic, and diagnosis cannot be made on a radiographic basis alone. The lesion appears as an expansile cystic mass that is usually unilocular, although it may be multilocular. As the lesion increases in size, there may be marked expansion and thinning of the cortex, resulting in a ballooning, blowout, honeycomb, or soap bubble appearance that is noticeably abnormal. If the lesion involves the region of the teeth, root resorption may be seen. The teeth may be displaced but remain vital.

Grossly, the specimen is soft reddish brown because of its rich blood supply, and it resembles a sponge filled with blood.

Differential Diagnosis (see p. 59)

The lesion can easily be mistaken for an odontogenic cyst or tumor, a central giant cell granuloma, a myxoma, a central hemangioma of bone, a giant cell lesion of hyperparathyroidism, cherubism, and even a low-grade metastatic carcinoma.

Laboratory Aids

Biopsy will demonstrate characteristic large spaces that are lined by flattened cells and filled with uncoagulated blood. The walls and septi consist of fibrous tissue containing variable amounts of fibroblasts, osteoid and immature bone permeated by foci of hemosiderin, and many multinucleated giant cells of the foreign body or osteoclastic type.

Treatment

Curettage has been the most frequent treatment for aneurysmal bone cyst of the jaws. Radiation therapy does not appear to be effective, and it may introduce the hazard of postradiation sarcoma. Radiation should be reserved for those cases in which surgical removal is not feasible. The recommended dosage appears to be somewhere between a minimum of 600 rads and a maximum of 2000 rads. The risk of postradiation sarcoma increases with larger or excessive dosages of radiation.

It is our opinion that aneurysmal bone cyst of the jaws is best treated by enucleation, curettage, and filling of the defect with bone chips. Cryosurgery could be applied before placement of the bone chips, especially in case of incomplete removal of the lesion.

Angioedema (1B22)

Angioedema (angioneurotic edema) is a well-demarcated, sessile edema of the dermal submucosa caused by an immediate type of hypersensitivity reaction to an allergen, such as a drug, that has either contacted the skin, been ingested, or been injected. Penicillin, the sulfonamides, barbiturates, and certain tranquilizers are the most frequent offenders.

Clinical Features

Within minutes after contact with the allergen, a rapidly developing, painless swelling of the affected part appears and persists for 24 hours or even for several days. The lips, the periorbital skin, and the tongue are most commonly affected. An itching or burning sensation may precede the swelling. The edematous tissue is normal in color, is of nonpitting consistency, and has a fairly well demarcated contour. The lymph nodes are not usually palpable. Complications may arise if the inflammation affects the glottis or the larynx (Quincke's edema).

Differential Diagnosis (see p. 10)

An idiopathic and a hereditary form of angioedema are known, the latter being due to a lack of the inhibitor of the first component of the complement cascade.

Laboratory Aids

For the hereditary type, a number of laboratory tests are available to demonstrate the inhibitor of the first component of the complement.

Treatment

The allergen should be identified whenever possible. Antihistamines and adrenaline may be administered for acute episodes involving the glottis.

Ankyloglossia (2E60)

Ankyloglossia, which is generally partial, is a congenital shortening of the lingual frenulum such that it extends from the anterior ventral surface of the tongue to the anterior lingual mandibular gingiva. This abnormal frenulum is very thick and interferes with normal extension of the tongue. In some families this condition is inherited as an autosomal dominant.

Clinical Features

The thick frenulum may produce diastemas between the mandibular central incisors. The tongue mobility is impaired, but speech, phonation, and deglutition are within normal limits. Ankyloglossia seems to affect males more often than females. Its frequency has been estimated at 1 in 400 individuals in the population in general. Cases of complete attachment of the tongue to the floor of the mouth or to the alveolar gingiva are extremely rare but have been reported.

Differential Diagnosis (see p. 25)

In the oral-facial-digital syndrome, the tongue may present several lateral frenula and is generally cleft. Ankyloglossia also has been seen in association with the cleft lip-palate and congenital lip pits syndrome (1C26).

Laboratory Aids

None.

Treatment

In extreme cases, debridement by surgical procedure can free the tongue. In such cases extreme care must be taken, because the frenulum is traversed by a large artery and a vein.

Apert's Syndrome (1A3, 1A4, and 1A5; 3E58)

Apert's syndrome is a form of craniosynostosis consisting of turribrachycephaly and syndactyly of hands and feet. The incidence is 1 in 160,000 live births with an equal distribution between sexes. The syndrome is transmitted as an autosomal dominant condition, but the majority of cases are sporadic. An advanced paternal age effect has been demonstrated.

Clinical Features

The middle third of the face appears flat and underdeveloped, producing a relative mandibular prognathism. The nose is sometimes small and shaped somewhat like a parrot's beak. Hypertelorism and strabismus are often noted. The orbits are flattened, and the eyes are proptosed. High-arched palate, occasionally with a marked median furrow, is a frequent finding. Cleft palate or bifid uvula is found in 25% of patients with Apert's syndrome. Hypoplastic maxilla and relative mandibular prognathism with an irregular positioning of the teeth is a constant finding. Crowding of the teeth leads to a marked thickening of the alveolar process. The pointed palate causes protrusion of the middle portion of the upper lip. Most patients have an intelligence below normal. The cranium has a characteristic oxycephalic appearance with temporal and frontal bulging. The forehead is steep and the occipital region is flat. Both hands and feet present symmetrical syndactyly that varies from partial skin fusion to true progressive osseous syndactyly of metacarpals, metatarsals, and phalanges. When the three middle fingers are completely fused, there is often a common nail that gives the hand the appearance of a mitten (mid-digital hand mass).

Differential Diagnosis (see pp. 9, 39)

The other types of acrocephalosyndactyly, Saethre-Chotzen's syndrome, and Crouzon's syndrome should be considered in the differential diagnosis.

Laboratory Aids

None known.

Treatment

None.

Ascher's Syndrome (1B20)

Ascher's syndrome is composed of blepharochalasis, double lip, and possibly thyroid enlargement. The condition is of unknown etiology, although vasomotor instability, hormonal dysfunction, and autosomal dominant inheritance have been suggested.

Clinical Features

The characteristic facies is best appreciated during smiling or talking. It is characterized by sagging eyelids and thick double upper lip. The skin of the upper lids is markedly thin and atrophic. Episodes similar to angioneurotic edema are frequent. The enlargement of the eyelids and lips may occur simultaneously. The lower lids are rarely, if ever, affected. The upper lip is characterized by a horizontal duplication, seen only when the patient smiles or talks. The double lip can be present from infancy and is located in the mucosa of the upper lip. The lower lip is almost always normal. Thyroid enlargement is variable and not associated with toxic symptoms. Several cases of Ascher's syndrome without thyroid enlargement have been seen.

Differential Diagnosis (see p. 9)

Double lip, the Melkersson-Rosenthal's syndrome, lip lymphedema, goiter, and vascular neoplasia of the lips should be considered in the differential diagnosis.

Laboratory Aids

None.

Treatment

Corrective surgery of the upper lip can be accomplished if the patient so desires.

Aspirin Burn (2B15)

Intraoral burns can be produced by a variety of chemical and physical agents, such as acids, certain medicaments, smoking, hot foods, or radiation. Probably the most frequent chemical burn is caused by the direct (contact) application of an aspirin tablet to the oral mucusa.

Clinical Features

Aspirin burns are essentially first-degree burns. The affected mucosal surface presents a rounded area of ulceration, corresponding to the shape of the tablet, with a marked necrotic halo. A whitish pseudomembrane, formed by epithelial sloughing, generally appears, at the periphery of the lesion, 24 hours after the initial application of the tablet. Pain is an accompanying feature. The lesion may occur in any area of the oral mucosa but generally is in the vicinity of a painful tooth. The burn is produced by the acetylsalicylic acid contained in the tablet.

Healing occurs within a week, generally without scarring. Markedly large lesions leave a residual scar. Secondary infection, especially in those patients with poor oral hygiene, is a possible complication and might alter the prognosis.

Differential Diagnosis (see p. 22)

All the white lesions affecting the oral mucosa should be considered, especially moniliasis and snuff dipper's pouch. Traumatic ulceration of various causes should also be considered. Squamous cell carcinoma, especially in older patients, should also be ruled out. The best diagnostic aid is a careful interrogation of the patient to ascertain the local use of aspirin.

Laboratory Aids

None.

Treatment

Rinsing with any mouth wash to maintain oral hygiene, thus preventing secondary infections.

Basal Cell Epithelioma (1A12)

Basal cell epithelioma, also called basal cell carcinoma, is a neoplasm derived from the basal cells in the epidermis or from the adnexal structures of the skin. This neoplasm usually does not meet the criteria of a malignant neoplasm, because it does not metastasize. Basal cell epithelioma grows by extension. Therefore, it is viewed as a locally aggressive lesion but not a truly malignant tumor.

Clinical Features

This lesion occurs essentially in the skin. It has never been reported inside the oral cavity, except as an extension of a tumor originally developing in the skin of the cheek. It is frequently seen in individuals who work outdoors, such as farmers and sailors, or in individuals who sunbathe the year around. It is also seen occasionally in persons exposed to large doses of radiation on the skin. The tumors can be single or multiple and generally are a few centimeters in diameter. The lesion is raised over the surface of the skin and occasionally presents a central depression. After a short period of growth it generally ulcerates in the center. Dilated blood vessels at the periphery of the lesion are also seen. The condition is not painful. The lesion tends to bleed very easily owing to increased vascularization. If untreated, a lesion can reach very large sizes with marked destruction of the affected areas. On the face lesions are sometimes associated with areas of trauma, occurring sometimes in individuals who wear eyeglasses (1A12), either on the infraorbital region or on the ear. Multiple lesions can be distributed not only over the face, but also throughout the trunk and extremitites.

Differential Diagnosis (see p. 9)

A great variety of lesions in this case should be considered, among them pigmented verruca vulgaris, squamous cell carcinoma of the skin, senile keratosis, keratoacanthoma, and some other lesions of interest primarily to the dermatologist. In the case of multiple lesions, the multiple nevoid basal cell carcinoma syndrome must be ruled out (1A11).

Laboratory Aids

Biopsy of the lesion, which generally should be performed by a dermatologist, will demonstrate the nature of the process.

Treatment

Basal cell carcinomas can be treated by several means, among them surgery, electrocauterization, and cryosurgery. Treatment is essentially in the hands of the dermatologist.

Bell's Palsy (1A7)

This is a unilateral paralysis of the muscles of facial expression due to ischemia of the facial nerve with some degree of myelin degeneration. The condition is predominantly idiopathic, though trauma and cold stress have been implicated. Some familial cases have been found. Neoplasms or surgical division of the facial nerve may induce this condition. Bell's palsy can also be associated with viral infections, as is the case with herpes zoster (Ramsey-Hunt's syndrome). In these cases a vesicular eruption can be observed in the auricular canal, as well as in the oral mucosa, following the distribution of the affected nerve.

Clinical Features

The patient is unable to wrinkle the forehead, to screw up the orbicularis oculi, or to blink. Consequently, foreign bodies may become lodged in the eye and tears may be abundant. The patient cannot smile on the side affected, and loss of muscle tone in the lip results in saliva running out of the corner of the mouth and in the development of angular cheilitis. Taste sensation may be altered on the anterior two-thirds of the affected side of the tongue. In the idiopathic form the prognosis is good. The paralysis is frequently transient and lasts, at most, about 3 months. Women are more commonly affected.

Differential Diagnosis (see p. 9)

Absence of gustatory sweating eliminates auriculotemporal syndrome. The history is inconsistent with jaw-winking syndrome. Absence of edema and lingua plicata eliminates the Melkersson-Rosenthal's syndrome.

Laboratory Aids

Electromyographic studies are useful.

Treatment

Since spontaneous remission is anticipated, treatment is not generally required in the idiopathic form. Surgical nerve decompression within the first 3 months may restore function; cortisone has been found to be beneficial.

Benign Migratory Glossitis and Migratory Mucositis (2A11; 2C36)

Benign migratory glossitis (geographic tongue) is a benign inflammatory condition in which areas of superficial keratin and filiform papillae desquamate. Its cause is unknown. Multifactorial polygenic inheritance has been suggested.

Clinical Features

The lesions are usually multiple and appear as pink to red denuded areas with white serpiginous borders. Intraepithelial inflammation at the white borders is followed by loss and then healing of papillae in the red areas. Pain or a burning sensation may accompany lesions that have a prominent inflammatory component. Lesions occur on the dorsum of the tongue, although the lateral borders may be involved. Lesions have been observed to migrate from site to site. The fungiform papillae are not affected by the process.

The condition appears suddenly and persists for weeks, months, or even years. Spontaneous remissions and recurrences have been observed. The lesion is harmless. The rare mucosal counterpart, migratory mucositis (ectopic geographic tongue) (2A11), may occur simultaneously with geographic tongue or by itself.

Differential Diagnosis (see pp. 22, 24)

Diagnosis is rarely a problem; however, associated migratory mucositis and psoriasis should be looked for. Eruption due to drugs should also be considered.

Laboratory Aids

None.

Treatment

None.

Benign Mucous Membrane Pemphigoid (3D43, 3D44, and 3D45)

Benign mucous membrane pemphigoid is an autoimmune disorder, characterized by subepithelial bulla formation of the mucous membranes, especially the oral mucosa and the conjunctiva. The skin is affected occasionally.

Clinical Features

This is a chronic, nonfatal disease generally seen in older patients. Females are affected twice as frequently as males. The skin is the site of lesions in only 10% of the patients. The bullae can occur in any area of the oral mucosa and generally are few in number. Vesicles of various sizes, round and reddish pink, are the first manifestations of the disease; they last for 1 or 2 days and then rupture, leaving raw, bleeding surfaces. The ulcers are generally covered by a fibrinous exudate; peripheral epithelial slough is also seen. Erythema of the oral mucosa is a constant finding, generally persisting up to several weeks, even after the ulcers have healed. Oral lesions heal without scar formation.

The disorder is characterized by periods of exacerbation and remission. Development and healing of the lesions occur more slowly than in the other bullous disorders affecting the oral cavity. Repeated episodes in the eyes lead to cloudiness of the cornea, loss of cilia, and formation of fibrous cicatricial bands. Lack of tear secretion may lead to corneal damage with loss of vision.

Differential Diagnosis (see p. 38)

Pemphigus vulgaris, erythema multiforme, bullous lichen planus, aphthous stomatitis, desquamative gingivitis, Reiter's syndrome, bullous pemphigoid, and Behçet's syndrome should be differentiated.

Laboratory Aids

Biopsy will reveal subepithelial vesiculation. This finding is nonspecific but rules out pemphigus vulgaris. Direct immunofluorescence will demonstrate that immunoglobulins and complement are bound to the epithelial basement membrane. This finding is seen both within the lesions and in adjacent, clinically normal epithelium. Circulating antibodies to the basement membrane have been found in some patients with the disease. Indirect immunofluorescence will show similar findings.

Treatment

Maintenance doses of corticosteroids are successfully used in the treatment of this condition.

Bifid Uvula (3E59)

Bifid or cleft uvula is an incomplete form of cleft palate. This condition is observed in approximately 1 in 80 white individuals. The incidence is much higher in American Indians (from 1 in 9 to 1 in 14). In blacks the condition is rarely seen.

Clinical Features

Bifid uvula is characterized by a clefting of the uvula that can present several degrees, from very minor division at the tip of the uvula to a total separation of the uvula into two segments. The condition has no significant effect on phonation or deglutition.

Differential Diagnosis (see p. 39)

Differential diagnosis should include several well-known entities that might be associated with bifid uvula, such as mild cases of Pierre Robin's anomalad and hereditary progressive arthroophthalmopathy.

Laboratory Aids

None.

Treatment

None.

Blastomycosis, North American (1D43)

North American blastomycosis is a chronic infection caused by the organism *Blastomyces dermatitidis.* It is acquired through the respiratory tract and occasionally disseminated hematogenously to the bones and skin.

Clinical Features

This condition occurs most commonly in male farmers and laborers. The initial infection of the lungs spreads to the skin, where granulomatous lesions with superficial accumulations of pus form raised firm, subcutaneous nodules. Crusts may form that, when lifted, permit pus to exude. The center of the lesion may undergo ulceration and then heal to a thin depigmented atrophic scar. Bone lesions take the form of an osteomyelitis with superficial pus-discharging sinuses. The disease may affect the genitalia and the oral and nasal mucosae. General symptoms such as fever, malaise, and lassitude are seen in half the patients. The disease can have a poor prognosis, but some patients have only a mild progressive or even self-limiting condition.

Differential Diagnosis (see p. 11)

Other granulomatous disorders, as well as osteomyelitis of different origins, should be considered in the differential diagnosis.

Laboratory Aids

Smears of the pus mixed with 10% potassium hydroxide show large nucleated spores and occasional hyphae. The organism can be cultured on Sabouraud's medium.

Treatment

The condition is serious enough to warrant intravenous amphotericin B. Surgical drainage of abscesses and osteomyelitis is indicated.

Branchial Cleft Cyst (1E53)

The term "branchial cleft cyst" is reserved for lymphoepithelial cysts occurring on the neck. This lesion arises, most likely, from entrapment of salivary gland duct epithelium in lymph nodes.

Clinical Features

The cyst manifests itself as a lateral neck mass that may vary from 2 to 10 cm in diameter. This mass is fluctuant and painless, with a very slow growth. Palpation reveals that the cyst is not attached to the underlying structures. It is most frequently seen in patients 30 years of age or older.

Differential Diagnosis (see p. 12)

Lymphadenitis, lymphoma, carotid body tumor, and cystic hygroma should be included in the differential diagnosis.

Laboratory Aids

None.

Treatment

Surgical excision is the preferred treatment. The cyst may recur if improperly treated.

Buccal Exostosis (3B16; 5A1)

Buccal exostosis represents a developmental variation in normal bone contour, possibly inherited as an autosomal dominant.

Clinical Features

Multiple bone-hard nodular excrescences are found particularly on the buccal aspect of the maxillary alveolar mucosa bilaterally distributed above the mucogingival junction. The condition is more common in men than women and is asymptomatic. The only complication may arise with toothbrush trauma or denture wearing.

Differential Diagnosis (see pp. 36, 59)

Multiple osteomas generally associated with Gardner's syndrome need to be considered in the differential diagnosis.

Laboratory Aids

None.

Treatment

Surgical excision is indicated if a prosthesis needs to be placed in the area.

Calcifying Epithelial Odontogenic Tumor (5B24)

Calcifying epithelial odontogenic tumor, also known as Pindborg's tumor, is a rare, locally invasive neoplasm most commonly found associated with an unerupted tooth.

Clinical Features

The lesion most frequently (70% of the time) presents in the premolar-molar region of the mandible as a diffuse swelling involving the lower border. The tumor is very rare, but males around 40 years of age appear to be slightly more frequently affected than the general population. Although the tumor is somewhat less aggressive than ameloblastoma, it can be locally invasive, and extraosseous varieties have been reported. In general, it can be said that Pindborg's tumor has the same clinical characteristics and behavior as ameloblastoma. Radiographically, the lesion is multilocular with a poorly defined honeycomb appearance. It appears to be growing between the roots of adjacent teeth. An unerupted tooth may be associated. Speckled calcification is evident in the majority of the cases, distinguishing this tumor from ameloblastoma, which does not calcify.

Differential Diagnosis (see p. 60)

Ameloblastoma should be differentiated.

Laboratory Aids

The histopathology of these tumors may be widely varied but is characterized by polyhedral epithelial cell masses that undergo intracellular calcification. The result is calcific aggregates that may grow to become radiographically visible. The epithelial component resembles the reduced enamel epithelium.

Treatment

Local block resection of the mandible with preservation of the lower border, if possible, is the treatment of choice. Bone grafting may be necessary.

Candidiasis, Acute Pseudomembranous (2B17; 2E50)

Acute pseudomembranous candidiasis (moniliasis, or thrush) is an acute superficial infection by *Candida albicans* on the surface epithelium of mucous membranes and occasionally the skin. *Candida albicans* is a normal commensal yeastlike fungus. Under conditions of altered host resistance, it can give rise to a variety of acute, chronic, and systemic infections.

Clinical Features

The acute pseudomembranous infection is found most frequently in the oral mucosa of newborn infants, presenting usually as curdlike, white plaques that are easily removed, leaving a raw, painful, bleeding surface. A maternal vaginitis usually is the source. The disorder may arise when the ecology of the normal oral flora is upset by broad-spectrum antibiotics, in patients on corticosteroid therapy, in patients with diabetes mellitus, and in patients with Addison's disease with or without hypoparathyroidism.

Any area of the oral cavity can be affected. The patient generally complains of a burning sensation and a metallic or altered taste. The affected area will present as a combination of white pseudomembrane formation and erythematous ulcerated areas. The pseudomembranous patches are easily peeled off.

Infection of the gastrointestinal and respiratory tracts and systemic spread to internal organs may occur as a terminal event in patients with primary or secondary immune deficiencies.

Differential Diagnosis (see pp. 22, 25)

Any disease capable of producing white patches may occasionally mimic acute pseudomembranous candidiasis, especially in the adult. Leukoplakia, lichen planus, genokeratoses, syphilitic mucous patches, and aspirin burn should be considered. Squamous cell carcinoma is frequently associated with secondary *Candida* infection.

Laboratory Aids

The virulent form of the organism is identified as branching pseudohyphae and spores in smears by using a 10% solution of potassium hydroxide or in sections by fungal stains such as MacManus PAS. The organism is easily cultured on Sabouraud's medium. Cultures will demonstrate the fungal colonies in 24 to 48 hours.

Treatment

The infection responds to local antifungal agents such as mycostatin and amphotericin B. The length of the treatment depends on the degree of the involvement and the resistance of the fungus to the antifungal agent.

Candidiasis, Mucocutaneous (1C32; 2E51)

Mucocutaneous candidiasis (moniliasis) is a generalized infection of mucous membranes and skin by *Candida albicans* secondary to an immune deficiency. Similarly, endocrine abnormalities such as idiopathic hypoparathyroidism and/or Addison's disease may predispose to this condition.

Clinical Features

The mucosal lesions may take the form of an acute pseudomembranous candidiasis (2B17; 2E50) or may be a firm, adherent leukoplakia of the mucous membranes. Cracks and fissures of the lips are surrounded by hypertrophic candidal granulomas (as in 1C32). Perianal, vulvovaginal, and penile lesions may also be present. The scalp is rarely affected. Skin lesions in the intertriginous zones may be red, weeping, intensely itchy, and painful. Nail lesions are most common; the soft skin at the base and sides of the nails becomes red, swollen, and painful (paronychia), and the nails become brown and eroded at the edge and present transverse ridges.

Differential Diagnosis (see pp. 10, 25)

The duration of the condition is inconsistent with angioedema or a drug allergy. Various biochemical and immunologic assays would be required to discriminate the underlying endocrine or immune defect.

Laboratory Aids

Laboratory aids are the same as for acute pseudomembranous candidiasis.

Treatment

Nystatin or amphotericin B creams or ointments may be applied to the skin. Systemic antifungal therapy is also indicated.

Caries, Dental
(4B18 and 4B19; 4C28; 4C33; 4D44 and 4D45)

Dental plaque, a virtually invisible colony of bacteria that forms a sticky, gelatinous mass of extracellular polysaccharide polymers, is thought to be the etiologic agent of dental caries. The production of this cariogenic plaque is favored by a preponderance of sucrose in the diet. Sucrose is easily biodegradable and favors the growth of certain microorganisms that use the high energy of the disaccharide bond for their metabolism and, more importantly, for the elaboration of the extracellular polysaccharide polymers. Several oral bacteria appear to have the capacity to produce a viscous retentive plaque. Within this plaque, fermentation reactions yield acid from rapid anaerobic catabolism of refined dietary carbohydrates to lactic acid. This and other acids so produced decalcify the enamel of the tooth. The plaque also isolates an area of increasing acidity from the bicarbonate buffering capacity of saliva. Hence, any disease, drug, or therapy that gives a dry mouth contributes to caries.

Clinical Features

The early lesion of dental caries is a white spot of decalcification on the enamel surface (as in 4C28). This is followed by cavitation, which usually occurs on the smooth surfaces of the interproximal areas, in pits and fissures of the occlusal surfaces, or at the gingival margin. (The case illustrated in 4C28 is unusual in that the distribution was determined by the tooth surfaces covered by orthodontic bands.) Penetration of the enamel is followed by a more rapid decalcification of the underlying dentin. The dentin becomes softened when its tubules are invaded by colonies of bacteria. The decalcification process may provoke pain; however, dental caries at this stage is generally a painless disease and can only be detected in pits and fissures and interproximal areas as a yielding catch to a sharp dental explorer or by radiography. Further decalcification and destruction of the protein matrix of the dentin undermines the enamel, which subsequently breaks down to form clinically obvious cavities (4B18 and 4B19, 4C28). A clinically visible cavity is a fairly advanced carious lesion. Dental caries progresses to involve the pulp with acute or chronic inflammation, death of the pulp, periapical abscess, periapical granuloma, periapical sinus, or apical radicular cyst.

The importance of sucrose as an occupational hazard in candy makers is illustrated in 4B18 and 4B19. Materia alba (i.e., food debris and dental plaque) is obvious as white collections on the tooth surfaces, and the radiograph demonstrates the extensive punched-out lesions that are produced by rampant caries (4B19). This case should be compared with that illustrated in 4D44 and 4D45, where sucrose in soft drinks has caused rampant caries. With the withdrawal of the sucrose and further treatment, these carious lesions have undergone some degree of arrest. Arrested caries is heavily pigmented and leathery in consistency (as in 4C33).

Differential Diagnosis (see pp. 48, 49)

The clinical appearance of caries is typical enough not to warrant a differential diagnosis. Systemic causes, such as Sjögren's syndrome (4C31) and others that could be associated with marked xerostomia, should be ruled out in cases of rampant caries in older individuals.

Laboratory Aids

Various microbiologic tests and tests for acid production are available as criteria of patients at risk for dental caries. However, the best prognosticator appears to be the patient's recent history of dental caries.

Treatment

Carious dentin and enamel are removed, and the cavities are restored with obtundent, sealing, and bacteriocidal cements and covered with silver amalgam or gold or tooth-colored composite materials.

Prevention of further dental caries is a joint effort involving the dentist or dental hygienist and the patient. The professional must educate the patient in proper diet (especially in the need for avoiding snacks and beverages containing sucrose), in toothbrushing and flossing techniques, and in the importance of regular prophylaxis and polishing by the hygienist. The patient must follow through on these preventive measures.

Caries, Dental, Radiation (4D46)

This form of dental caries is secondary to the dryness of the mouth (xerostomia) caused by the destruction of salivary gland tissue that occurs after treatment with ionizing radiation. Saliva seems to offer several potential mechanisms for protecting teeth against caries—specific and nonspecific bacteriocidal factors, buffering capacity, lubrication, and others.

Clinical Features

Xerostomia may be of insidious onset. The patient complains of tacky saliva and a need to drink frequently. The progress of the caries is rampant, involving primarily the cervical margins of the teeth but also the incisal surfaces of the anterior and cuspid teeth. Whole crowns may be destroyed (as in 4D46). There is some controversy as to whether dental hard tissues are directly affected by radiation. It has been suggested that the enamel and dentin become more brittle and dehydrated and consequently more prone to the development of lesions. The main hazard of postradiation caries is, however, the potential of dental infection to the underlying bone. Bone vasculature is readily damaged by irradiaton, and infection of this damaged bone can lead to a protracted osteomyelitis termed osteoradionecrosis. Such infection can arise if teeth are removed after irradiation. Healing of the tooth sockets is delayed. The bone dies easily and forms sequestra. Osteoradionecrosis of the jaws is extremely painful and runs a protracted course. Sequestration is slow, and whole segments of the mandible or maxilla may die or be sloughed.

Differential Diagnosis (see p. 49)

The differential diagnosis should include those other conditions associated with xerostomia or rampant caries.

Laboratory Aids

None.

Treatment

Patients who are to undergo radiation for the treatment of cancer of the head and neck must have dental and radiographic evaluations to determine whether it is necessary to extract all of the remaining teeth. If the patient has good oral hygiene and a dentition free of caries and other dental abnormalities, and if the radiation dose is considered unlikely to obliterate the salivary gland tissue, the teeth may be retained with a regimen of dental checkups, fluoride gel treatments at regular intervals, and regular prophylaxis. Otherwise, the teeth should be removed with minimal surgical trauma, the crest of the bone should be trimmed, and the alveolar mucosa should be approximated over the tooth sockets with sutures. In view of the hazards of the development of radiation caries and osteoradionecrosis, the predominant dental opinion is against the use of radiotherapy for malignant oral neoplasms.

Caries, Dental, Secondary to Sjögren's Syndrome (4C31)

Dental caries can occur secondary to xerostomia accompanying Sjögren's syndrome, which consists of keratoconjunctivitis sicca, xerostomia, and rheumatoid arthritis. The syndrome is thought to have an autoimmune pathogenesis in which salivary and lacrimal gland tissue is destroyed by lymphocytic infiltration.

Clinical Features

The patient has a dry mouth and the salivary glands may or may not be enlarged. The tongue may be fissured. Dental caries is predominantly cervical but can also affect the incisal edges and may obliterate the crowns of teeth (as in 4C31). The patient may complain of sensations of something in the eyes, burning sensations, or inability to produce tears. Swallowing may be difficult, and patients increase their fluid intake. Rheumatoid disease is expressed as erosive arthritis, subcutaneous nodules, and splenomegaly. The salivary glands, especially the parotid, may be enlarged. Lymphomas may develop in some patients.

Differential Diagnosis (see p. 48)

The differential diagnosis can include other sources of xerostomia, such as radiation. Rampant caries of other origin should also be considered.

Laboratory Aids

Biopsy of minor mucous salivary glands may be of assistance in diagnosis. Serum electrophoresis will show hypergammaglobulinemia.

Treatment

Artificial saliva and tears may relieve symptoms. Therapy for rheumatoid arthritis should be arranged. Oral hygiene, topical fluorides, and diet counseling should be applied to arrest the progress of dental caries.

Cellulitis, Acute (4E58 and 4E59)

Acute cellulitis is a poorly circumscribed inflammation of the soft tissues resulting from infection by pyogenic microorganisms, particularly streptococci. Periapical abscesses and osteomyelitis are accompanied by an acute cellulitis.

Clinical Features

The patient is moderately ill and has malaise, fever, and lassitude. The tissues are tensely swollen and feel indurated (brawny edema). The overlying skin may be reddish or purplish. As a complication, the infection may track along tissue planes and form focal abscesses in peripheral sites. Lymphadenitis is usually present. The nodes are very tender to palpation.

Differential Diagnosis (see p. 50)

Depending on the location, the differential diagnosis could include several types of neoplasia, including leukemias and specific granulomatous inflammations among the most frequent.

Laboratory Aids

None.

Treatment

The infection will have a prompt resolution if treated with antibiotics and removal of the offending tooth or teeth.

Cheek Biting (2B24)

Cheek biting (morsicatio buccarum) results in an irregular white patch on the oral mucosa. Because cheek biting can occur during sleep, some patients with lesions are unaware of their cause.

Clinical Features

The change occurs only in those areas of the oral mucosa that can be reached by teeth. The affected area becomes corrugated and white with a typical macerated surface. Occasionally, a small hematoma may be seen. The lesion will disappear if the patient abandons the habit.

Differential Diagnosis (see p. 48)

The differential diagnosis should include lesions induced by mechanical irritation and snuff dipper's pouch.

Laboratory Aids

None.

Treatment

None, but the patient should be advised to abandon the habit.

Cheilitis, Angular (1C33)

Angular cheilitis (also known as cheilitis or perlèche) consists of erosions, crusts, and radiating erythematous fissures at the labial commissures, associated with *Candida albicans* and some bacteria. The condition may be associated with vitamin B-group deficiencies.

Clinical Features

In patients with a skin fold at the angle between the upper and lower lips which is constantly wet with saliva, the skin becomes macerated, cracks, and erodes. This may induce a small nodular granulomatous reaction that contributes to the persistence of the condition (1C32). It is most common in women whose dentures have reduced vertical dimension and who do not maintain the physiologic tone of the circumoral tissues.

Differential Diagnosis (see p. 10)

Commissural lip pits are readily distinguished from this condition because they are noninflamed, blind-ended pits at the commissural vermilion border.

Laboratory Aids

Smears or cultures for identification of *Candida albicans* or other organisms are recommended. Dietary analysis should be considered to identify a vitamin deficiency.

Treatment

This is generally a chronic or recurrent condition that improves with new dentures and/or antifungal therapy. The nodular reaction may require careful surgical removal. Vitamin A therapy may be beneficial.

Cheilitis, Chronic Actinic (1D37)

Chronic actinic cheilitis (or solar keratosis), which results from prolonged exposure to sunlight, is characterized by a diffuse gray-white scaling of the vermilion border of the lower lip and commissures. The changes are seen most frequently in individuals who have an outdoor occupation.

Clinical Features

Chronic actinic cheilitis manifests as a diffuse, patchy, gray-white scale on the vermilion border of the lower lip due principally to hyperkeratinization of the epithelium and underlying elastosis of the dermis. Pigmentary and angiomatous changes also are apparent secondary to exposure to sunlight. If ulceration (as in 1D37) or induration is present, malignant or premalignant changes should be suspected. This condition may remain stationary for several years but is nevertheless thought to be a precancerous one.

Differential Diagnosis (see p. 11)

Candidiasis rarely if ever presents in this form on the lips. Leukoplakia is merely a descriptive term, and squamous cell carcinoma would be a histologic decision in this instance.

Laboratory Aids

Biopsy is important to determine the histologic appearance of the lesion. Senile elastosis may be apparent in the dermis.

Treatment

Prophylactic sunscreening creams such as zinc oxide ointment are used. Consideration should be given to the use of 5-fluorouracil.

Cheilitis Glandularis (1B21)

Cheilitis glandularis is an uncommon diffuse enlargement and eversion of the lower lip, with inflammation of the minor mucous salivary glands of unknown etiology.

Clinical Features

The lower lip is swollen and everted. The orifices of the minor mucous salivary glands are red, inflamed, and dilated and may secrete a viscous mucus. Progress to a deeper suppurative inflammation with abscesses and fistulae can occur (cheilitis glandularis apostematosa). The condition is thought on occasions to precede squamous cell carcinoma. Young adult males are most frequently affected.

Differential Diagnosis (see p. 9)

Actinic cheilitis (1D37) should be considered. Angioedema is acute in onset and of transient duration; no surface changes are present (1B22). The distinction from cheilitis granulomatosa is difficult without biopsy. If the patient has a history of facial edema, facial paralysis, and tongue changes, the Melkersson-Rosenthal's syndrome should be considered.

Laboratory Aids

None.

Treatment

None. Avoidance of chronic exposure to sun and tobacco are to be encouraged. Antibiotic and surgical treatment is required if the lesions progress to suppuration.

Chemical Burn (1B24)

A great number of acid and caustic medications are capable of producing intraoral burns. The case illustrated here represents an example of a burn with silver nitrate.

Clinical Features

These burns are generally of first degree. They rarely reach second degree. The burns are generally produced as a result of a caustic agent being used, generally to cauterize a previous area of ulceration such as a minor aphthous ulcer. Sometimes they are of iatrogenic origin, accidentally produced by the dentist using some of these caustic agents during dental procedures. The lesion can vary in size depending upon the amount of chemical spilled or the manner in which it was used. It can affect any area of the oral cavity and usually presents as a whitish, charred area. In the case of caustic agents, pain is usually absent, because the nerve terminals are also destroyed. Healing occurs within 1 or 2 weeks, and generally there is no complication or scar tissue formation.

Differential Diagnosis (see p. 10)

Other white lesions affecting the oral mucosa should be considered, especially moniliasis. Traumatic ulceration should also be considered. Burns produced by silver nitrate must be differentiated from mucous patches in secondary syphilis. Careful interrogation of the patient to ascertain local use of chemicals is an important aid in establishing the final diagnosis.

Laboratory Aids

None.

Treatment

None.

Cherubism (5B13 and 5B14)

Cherubism is a familial multilocular bone disease that almost exclusively affects the jaws. The condition is inherited in an autosomal dominant mode with variable expressivity and incomplete penetrance in females. Cherubism is not considered to be a form of fibrous dysplasia of the jaws.

Clinical Features

The syndrome begins to manifest itself between the ages of 18 months and 4 years as a painless swelling, the affected individual being normal at birth. Generally, involvement is bilateral, but unilateral cases have occasionally been reported. Maxilla and mandible can be affected at the same time, but the maxilla is less often involved. The maxilla is most frequently affected in the area of the antrum and the tuberosity. Involvement of the orbital floor will produce upward displacement of the eye, exposing a characteristic rim of sclera beneath the iris. This, associated with the bilateral swelling, gives the typical cherubic appearance. Ocular hypertelorism is an almost constant feature. The bone is replaced by fibrous connective tissue with multinucleated giant cells. This produces displacement of primary teeth as well as abortive formation or absence of permanent molar teeth. Radiographically, the bone has a soap bubble appearance generally extending bilaterally from the molar region to the angle and ramus of the mandible. The condyle is never affected. Severe cases may evidence total involvement of the mandible. The jaws increase rapidly in size until about puberty, when the swelling tends to remain stationary and then progressively disappears. After the age of 20 the only remaining radiographic evidence is scattered areas of slightly increased bone density. Severe cases may exhibit a grotesque appearance with complications in mastication, deglutition, respiration, and speech.

Differential Diagnosis (see p. 59)

Odontogenic tumors (i.e., ameloblastoma), fibrous dysplasia, primary and metastatic tumors of the jaws, aneurysmal bone cysts, and central giant cell tumor of the jaws should be considered in the differential diagnosis.

Laboratory Aids

Serum alkaline phosphatase levels may occasionally be elevated during the active phase of the disease.

Treatment

None.

Chicken Pox (1B14 and 1B15)

Chicken pox (varicella) is a contagious disease produced by a DNA virus. The disease generally occurs in children between the ages of 2 and 8 years. The virus remains latent in the dorsal root sensory ganglia, and it can be reactivated by various stresses producing shingles (herpes zoster) during adulthood.

Clinical Features

Within 10 to 21 days after exposure to the virus, usually via other children with chicken pox, the patient presents with mild symptoms characterized by slightly increased body temperature and malaise. Within 12 to 36 hours after onset of these symptoms, a rash appears, generally on the trunk. This rash is formed by red macules that progress to papules and eventually become vesicles. Marked pruritus is an almost constant clinical finding. Progressively, the lesions extend to the skin of the face. Intraoral lesions also occur; they are secondary to the skin vesicles and can be located almost anywhere in the oral cavity. Vesicles continue to appear through the first 3 or 4 days after initiation of the rash. After 7 to 10 days these vesicles will crust, indicating the beginning of the healing period. These lesions generally heal without scarring, but occasionally some individual lesion may leave a small, permanent scar. Complications can occur in the form of secondary bacterial infection for skin lesions. Some of these complications are dissemination to other organs as well as encephalitis due to invasion of the central nervous system. Chicken pox can be a deadly condition if it occurs in patients who are immunosuppressed, in patients who have an immune deficiency, or in patients who are leukemic.

Differential Diagnosis (see p. 9)

The clinical characteristics and epidemiologic nature of the disease make it a very easy one to diagnose. Nevertheless, early skin lesions can be confused with smallpox, dermatitis herpetiforme, eczema, and even impetigo. Oral lesions should be differentiated from herpes simplex, and if varicella occurs in adults one should not forget pemphigus vulgaris. Herpes zoster is generally characterized by a linear effusion of vesicles that follow the distribution of a terminal branch of a peripheral nerve.

Laboratory Aids

Laboratory tests are rarely used, but one could include cytologic examination of scrapings of the vesicle, showing large giant cells with inclusion bodies. These findings are also shared by herpes simplex. Furthermore, antibody titers can be read in sera of affected patients.

Treatment

The condition requires bed rest, diet as tolerated, and prevention of secondary infection. It is important to recognize that for immunosuppressed children with no previous history of varicella the condition could have a fatal outcome. These cases are treated with zoster immune globulin (ZIG) in order to prevent or modify the clinical course of chicken pox.

Cleft Lip, Cleft Palate, and Submucous Palatal Cleft (1B19; 1C26; 3E57; 3E58)

Clefting of the lip and/or palate is a congenital anomaly produced by lack of fusion of the embryonal processes involved in the formation of these anatomical areas. These abnormalities are considered multifactorial in origin. Some very well known and defined syndromes that are inherited in various ways are known to be associated with clefting. In these particular cases patients need to be carefully identified due to the fact that genetic counseling will be different from that of isolated clefting, which is not associated with inherited conditions.

Clinical Features

Clefting may involve only the upper lip or it may also complicate the nose as well as the hard and soft palates. Isolated cleft palate may be limited to the uvula (3E59). Also, it can be manifested as submucous cleft of the soft palate (as in 3E57). The most frequent clinical combination (representing about 50% of the cases) is that of cleft lip and cleft palate. Cleft lip represents 25% of the cases, and isolated cleft palate represents the remaining 25%. Cleft lip can be unilateral, in which case it is most frequently (70% of the time) observed on the left side. It can be bilateral, with the extreme case being bilateral cleft lip and palate.

Cleft lip with or without cleft palate is considered a single entity, and it represents about 1 in 1,000 births among Caucasians, 1.7 in 1,000 births among Orientals, and 1 in 2,500 births among black Americans. The highest incidence — 3.6 in 1,000 live births — is observed among American Indians. Among whites, the more severe the defect, the larger the number of affected males. Among blacks, females show a higher incidence of clefts as compared to the population in general.

Isolated cleft palate is considered a different entity from cleft lip with or without cleft palate. This separation is justified on the basis of statistics regarding families with isolated cleft palate. They have no higher incidence of cleft lip than that of the population in general. Cleft palate occurs in about 1 in 2,000 live births among whites and 1 in 2,500 live births among blacks. It occurs twice as often in females as in males.

Submucous palatal cleft is considered a minor form of cleft palate (3E57). In this case, the soft palate is generally short and the patients have a nasal quality to their speech. Occasionally, this condition is associated with bifid uvula. Submucous palatal cleft is observed with a slight preponderance in males. The incidence in the general population is estimated at 1 in 1,200 persons. Risk for cleft can be seen in Table 2. The different types of clefting are associated with other congenital anomalies with the following frequencies: isolated cleft palate between 13% and 50% of the time; isolated cleft lip between 7% and 13% of the time; and cleft lip and palate between 2% and 11% of the time. Patients with clefting of the lip and palate will have altered speech as well as irregularities in number and position of teeth. Especially common are absence of lateral maxillary incisors and malposition of incisor and cuspid teeth.

Differential Diagnosis (see pp. 9, 10, 38, 39)

Essentially, the differential diagnosis is limited to the various types of clefting and to the ability to ascertain the mode of inheritance, if any.

Laboratory Aids

None.

Treatment

Surgical correction of the defect early in life is indicated.

Cleft Lip-Palate and Congenital Lip Pits Syndrome (1C26)

The syndrome of cleft lip-palate and congenital lip pits is transmitted as an autosomal dominant condition with 80% penetrance for any component of the syndrome. The syndrome is seen with a frequency of about 1 in 75,000 to 100,000 live births and affects both sexes equally.

SHORT DESCRIPTIONS OF ORAL DISEASES

Table 2. Recurrence Risk for Clefts

	Cleft Lip and Palate (Percentage)	Cleft Palate (Percentage)
Normal parents:		
One affected child and no other children	4.0	3.5
One affected child and one normal child	4.0	3.0
Two affected children and no other children	14.0	13.0
One affected parent:		
No children	4.0	3.5
One affected child and no other children	12.0	10.0
One affected child and one normal child	10.0	9.0
Two affected children and no other children	25.0	24.0
Two affected parents:		
No children	35.0	25.0
One affected child and no other children	45.0	40.0
One affected child and one normal child	40.0	35.0
Two affected children and no other children	50.0	45.0

SOURCE: After M. Tolarova, *Acta Chir. Plast.* (Praha) 14: 234-35, 1972.

Clinical Features

Bilateral, symmetrical pits are located on the vermilion portion of the lower lip. These fistulas may be 3 mm or more in diameter or so small as barely to allow the introduction of a thin probe. The dimple may be circular or may present as a transverse slit. Rarely, they may be located at the apex of a nipplelike elevation. These depressions often exude saliva, spontaneously or upon pressure, because of their association with minor salivary glands. On microscopic sections, the pits have proven to be blind sinuses, descending through the orbicularis oris muscles.

In about 24% of cases, the pits are an isolated finding. In about 76% of cases, the pits are associated with cleft lip-palate. When associated with cleft lip-palate, the clefts are bilateral in over 80% of patients. A few cases have been reported in which there has been but a single pit. Adhesions between maxilla and mandible have also been noted. In the cases in which cleft lip is absent, the maxillary lateral incisors are missing or are hypoplastic (peg lateral). Miscellaneous oral findings have included ankyloglossia and cleft uvula.

Differential Diagnosis (see p. 10)

All the clefting syndromes should be included.

Laboratory Aids

None known.

Treatment

Corrective surgery is used at an early age for both cleft lip-palate and lip pits.

Cleidocranial Dysplasia (5A11 and 5A12)

Cleidocranial dysplasia consists of aplasia or hypoplasia of one or both clavicles, exaggerated development of the transverse diameter of the cranium, and delayed ossification of the fontanels. Cleidocranial dysplasia is transmitted in an autosomal dominant manner, although in approximately 50% of the cases it arises spontaneously, caused either by mutation or by a gene with poor penetrance.

Clinical Features

The face appears small, the nasal bridge is depressed, and the nose is broad at the base. The skull is brachycephalic with marked frontal, parietal, and occipital bossing. Fontanels and sutures remain open, often for life. Wormian bones are formed through secondary centers of ossification in the suture lines. The paranasal sinuses are often underdeveloped or absent.

Oral manifestations in the syndrome include supernumerary teeth and submucous or complete cleft palate. Pseudoanodontia is due to delayed eruption and impaction of deciduous, permanent, and supernumerary teeth. Cyst formation around these impacted teeth has been described by a number of investigators. In addition, the impacted teeth appear to lack a layer of cellular cementum. Probably the most prominent oral manifestation is in the extreme number of supernumerary teeth, which at times simulate a third dentition. Development of the premaxilla is poor, resulting in a false or relative prognathism.

Individuals with the syndrome are short in stature with long necks and narrow shoulders. The clavicles may be unilaterally or bilaterally aplastic or hypoplastic. Due to this bony defect, patients with the condition are able to approximate their shoulders in front of the chest.

Differential Diagnosis (see p. 59)

Pyknodysostosis, mandibuloacral dysplasia, and cleidofacial dysplasia should be included in the differential diagnosis.

Laboratory Aids

None known.

Treatment

Orthodontia is indicated to correct the multiple defects in tooth position. Corrective surgery of the palatal defect, when present, is also indicated. As in any other inherited disorder, proper genetic counseling is part of the treatment.

Congenital Epulis of the Newborn (3A4)

Congenital epulis of the newborn, also known as congenital granular cell myoblastoma, is a benign neoplasm which, as the name implies, is present at birth.

This lesion most likely is derived from striated muscle fibers. Some authors believe that it may be from nerve cell origin.

Clinical Features

The neoplasm is present at birth, as a rule in the maxillary midline, in the area to be occupied by the central maxillary incisors. A small number of cases have been observed to affect both the mandible and the maxilla. Eighty percent of affected infants to date have been females. This marked predilection for female infants is of unknown cause. The lesions can vary in size from a few millimeters to several centimeters in diameter, with the larger lesions appearing as rounded masses. Their color is similar to that of normal, adjacent mucosa. The tumors are generally pedunculated.

Differential Diagnosis (see p. 35)

Virtually the only other lesion that could be considered is neuroectodermal tumor of infancy, which can also be present at birth or appear shortly after birth in the same location (3A5) as congenital epulis of the newborn. These entities can be differentiated by their different colors and completely different histologies.

Laboratory Aids

Biopsy will demonstrate the nature of this lesion.

Treatment

Treatment consists of surgical excision. The neoplasm does not tend to recur.

Conoid Tooth (4A4)

Conoid tooth, or peg tooth, is an abnormality characterized by a change in shape of the crown of the tooth. This condition is most likely of multifactorial etiology.

Clinical Features

The tooth most frequently affected by this alteration is the lateral maxillary incisor, followed by the central mandibular incisors. There is no sex preference. Pegging of the maxillary lateral incisor occurs twice as often in the left side. In some families this condition is inherited as autosomal dominant.

Differential Diagnosis (see p. 47)

This change can be an isolated phenomenon restricted to one or two teeth or can be part of a systemic disorder, such as hypohidrotic ectodermal dysplasia, where not only conoid tooth but also hypodontia occurs. Supernumerary teeth in the anterior area as a rule present a conoid shape. Therefore, it is necessary to differentiate between a conoid supernumerary tooth and a conoid permanent tooth.

Laboratory Aids

None.

Treatment

Jacket crowns can be used in order to restore proper crown shape for these teeth.

Craniofacial Dysostosis (1A1 and 1A2)

Craniofacial dysostosis (Crouzon's syndrome) comprises cranial synostosis, bilateral exophthalmus with external strabismus, parrot-beaked nose, and relative mandibular prognathism with drooping lower lip. The syndrome is inherited as an autosomal dominant condition with almost complete penetrance. Sporadic cases with a negative family history, representing new mutations, are not infrequent.

Clinical Features

The facies is characterized by marked exophthalmus, due to shallow orbits. At times there is spontaneous luxation of the eyes. Ocular hypertelorism and hypoplastic maxilla are also constant findings. This last feature produces a marked relative mandibular prognathism and short upper lip. The cranium is brachycephalic with frontal bossing.

Oral manifestations include hypoplastic maxilla, a V-shaped palatal arch in contrast to the normal U-shaped arch, dental malocclusion, open bite, and partial clefting of the palate.

Eighty percent of affected individuals have optic nerve damage. Nystagmus is seen occasionally.

Differential Diagnosis (see p. 8)

Cleidocranial dysplasia and the acrocephalosyndactyly syndromes, as well as the craniosynostosis syndromes, should be included.

Laboratory Aids

None known.

Treatment

Corrective surgery can be used to ameliorate the facial appearance. The surgical procedure is not only complicated but also represents a high risk for the patient.

Cyclic Neutropenia (3A7 and 3A8)

Cyclic neutropenia is a periodic decrease of neutrophilic leukocytes in the peripheral blood. The clinical disease appears and regresses spontaneously, only to reappear in a cyclic pattern associated with the blood changes. An autosomal dominant mode of inheritance seems likely, although further evidence is needed to support this theory.

Clinical Features

Clinical manifestations generally begin in early childhood with mild fever, malaise, sore throat, oral involvement, and, in some cases, arthritis, headache, and cutaneous manifestations. Secondary infection is not of prime importance due to the short duration of the neutropenia.

Oral manifestations include severe ulcerative gingivitis or stomatitis or both. Occasionally, ulceration may be observed on the tongue, palate, and lip mucosa. Oral lesions are generally complicated by infection. Loss of alveolar bone results from repeated insults, leading to mobility and early exfoliation of teeth. Oral lesions may lead to partial or complete loss of teeth early in life.

Neutropenia usually lasts from 2 to 5 days. As the blood count returns to normal, the oral lesions regress. Ulcerations usually heal without scarring, but with successive attacks scarring may occur. The disease lasts throughout life. In some patients, spontaneous improvement may occur in adulthood. Cycles have an interval of approximately 21 to 27 days and occasionally range up to several months.

Differential Diagnosis (see p. 35)

Agranulocytosis, other blood dyscrasias, and recurrent aphthous ulceration should be considered. Other conditions producing premature loss of teeth should also be ruled out. The oral lesions in cyclic neutropenia have a marked similarity to those seen in Sutton's disease.

Laboratory Aids

Hematologic examination will show a marked decrease in neutrophils. Within 3 to 5 days the peak of the disease is reached, and for a period of 1 to 2 days neutrophils may be completely absent. Soon thereafter they reappear, and within 3 to 5 days the blood count and differential count are normal.

Treatment

There is no systemic treatment. If the patient's oral hygiene is properly maintained, the oral manifestations are reduced to a minimum or are absent.

Cystic Hygroma (1E55)

This multicystic mass is a developmental abnormality of lymphatic blood vessels. Cystic hygroma is thought to arise due to a failure of the lymphatic vessels in the neck area to drain in the central lymphatic system.

Clinical Features

The lesion is usually present at birth or appears shortly after birth. The classic location is the lateral aspect of the neck. The lesion is characterized by a slow, progressive growth. Occasional cases are associated with lymphangiomas of the tongue. Some cases undergo spontaneous regression. The lesions of cystic hygroma may reach grotesque proportions and can produce death by massive hemorrhage.

Differential Diagnosis (see p. 12)

The differential diagnosis should include a variety of neck masses, but this lesion is so characteristic, especially because of its congenital and/or neonatal appearance, that it is very rarely confused with any other entity.

Laboratory Aids

None.

Treatment

Treatment is essentially surgical. Danger of secondary infection prior to treatment is known to occur. It is advisable that this condition be treated as early as possible.

Dens in Dente (4D41)

Dens in dente, also known as dilated composite odontoma and dens invaginatus, is a developmental abnormality that most likely results from an invagination of the crown of a tooth bud before calcification of enamel and dentin occurs. The condition is of unknown etiology. In some families it is transmitted as an autosomal dominant.

Clinical Features

Dens in dente is most often observed in the lateral maxillary incisor but occasionally has been reported in the central maxillary incisor as well as in posterior teeth. There is no sex predilection. Dens in dente presents a great variation in clinical manifestations. Minor examples are characterized by an invagination of the lingual pit in the lateral maxillary incisor. Major examples are characterized by an invagination that starts in the crown and extends into the apical portion of the affected tooth, forming a tunnel of enamel inside of the dentin. In extreme cases the pulp is open to the oral cavity. Radiographically, dens in dente is easily diagnosed. The affected tooth generally has an abnormal crown shape; the severe forms are less commonly observed. The conditions, in all its various degrees, is quite frequent and in some studies is present in 5% of all patients.

Differential Diagnosis (see p. 49)

Radiographically, the condition is quite characteristic. Nevertheless, odontoma should be considered in the differential diagnosis, especially in extreme cases.

Laboratory Aids

None.

Treatment

Deep lingual pits in lateral incisors can be preventively obturated. The severe cases generally conduce to pulp necrosis with periapical pathology. In these cases, especially if the tooth is severely malformed, extraction is recommended. In less severe cases, endodontic treatment with proper restoration of crown shape can be attempted.

Dental Sinus (1D42; 1D44 and 1D45; 4B18 and 4B19; 4C33; 4D47 and 4D48)

The dental sinus (or dental fistula) is the tract through which purulent material from a dental septic focus deep in the bone, or around a tooth, drains into the skin or the oral mucous membrane.

Clinical Features

The dental sinus is usually single, appearing on the skin as a crusted erythematous nodule or pit (as in 1D42) or, owing to contraction of its walls, as a dimple-like fissure (as in 1D44). On the oral mucosa, the lesion may be an erythematous papule from which pus may be milked or a slight yellow elevation with an erythematous margin. Its site is dependent upon the path that offers the least resistance to the pus traveling from the apex of the offending tooth to the surface. The most common sites for cutaneous sinuses of dental origin are just below the inner canthus of the eye from the maxillary lateral incisor, cuspid, or first premolar tooth; just below the malar eminence from the maxillary premolars or first molar (as in 1D42); in the mental or submental area from the mandibular incisors, cuspid, or first premolar (as in 1D44); and in the lower border of the mandible and submandibular area from the lower mandibular molars and premolar teeth. Sinuses most commonly occur on the facial skin or the vestibular alveolar mucosa (as in 4C33; 4B18; 4D47) and occasionally on the palate and the floor of the mouth. The lymph nodes are rarely inflamed. The discharging sinus may persist for many years. If it becomes blocked, acute swelling and pain supervene.

Differential Diagnosis (see pp. 11, 47, 48, 49)

Actinomycosis and osteomyelitis are ruled out by lack of brawny edema.

Laboratory Aids

None. Smear of pus will rule out actinomycosis.

Treatment

Root canal treatment or extraction of the offending tooth is the treatment of choice. Excision of the fibrous scar tissue of the sinus tract may be necessary for cosmetic reasons. If the sinus has a cutaneous opening of long-standing duration, curettage or surgical debridement of the sinus tract is imperative in order to eliminate the epithelial lining that will interfere with normal healing.

Dentigerous Cyst (4E60)

The dentigerous or follicular cyst is a common type of odontogenic cyst that is always associated with the crown of an impacted or unerupted tooth, generally of the permanent dentition. The dentigerous cyst is thought to occur between the reduced enamel epithelium and the enamel after complete formation of the crown has taken place.

Clinical Features

The frequency of dentigerous cysts is difficult to ascertain. Some statistics show that 4% of patients with at least one unerupted tooth will have a dentigerous cyst. Some other statistics show that 37% of impacted mandibular third molars are associated with dentigerous cyst formation. Owing to its association with impacted teeth, the most frequent sites of occurrence are the mandibular third molar, the maxillary cuspid and third molar, and the second mandibular premolar. The condition can also be associated with any other unerupted tooth, including supernumerary teeth. Reports also have demonstrated that it can be associated with odontoma. The cyst growth is slow and eventually expands the cortical plates. The cyst can vary in size from a very small, almost imperceptible dilatation around the tooth crown to a cavity that occupies the entirety of the ascending ramus of the mandible. In cases in which the cyst reaches large proportions, facial asymmetry may be evident, and occasional paresthesia in the affected side due to compression of nerve terminals may be present.

Roentgenographically, it presents a characteristic image owing to the presence of the crown of the impacted tooth in the cystic cavity. The diagnosis of dentigerous cyst should be considered in those cases in which an impacted tooth crown is surrounded by a radiolucent space larger than 2 to 3 mm. In some cases the cyst will induce resorption of roots of neighboring teeth owing to pressure. In most cases the cyst embraces the whole crown, but in some cases the cyst can take a lateral position or even have a circumferential location in relation to the crown.

As a rule the cyst is unicameral, but occasionally it is multilocular, the different compartments communicating. In these cases, this cyst needs to be differentiated from ameloblastoma or odontogenic keratocyst. When the cyst develops in association with a maxillary third molar, it may invade the maxillary sinus. In such cases, different X rays should be taken in order to ascertain the real size of the cyst. The dentigerous cyst can also be multiple. In this instance it will most likely be associated with the multiple nevoid basal cell carcinoma syndrome. Transformation into an ameloblastoma or rarely into a squamous cell carcinoma is known to occur. Owing to these possible changes, all of these cysts must be submitted for histologic examination after surgical excision.

Differential Diagnosis (see p. 50)

The radiologic image is quite characteristic, but, nevertheless, one should consider ameloblastoma, aneurysmal bone cyst, odontogenic keratocyst, multiple nevoid basal cell carcinoma, and neoplastic pathology of bone that can arise in conjunction with a developing third molar.

Laboratory Aids

None.

Treatment

The treatment is surgery, but the surgical approaches depend on the size of the cyst. A small cyst can be treated by extraction of the impacted tooth and a very conservative surgical approach. Very large cysts, especially those which have produced resorption of large portions of the ascending ramus or the body of the mandible, are treated by marsupialization in order to avoid secondary fractures that can result from the great amount of bone loss.

Dentinal Dysplasia (4C36)

Dentinal dysplasia is a developmental abnormality of dentin inherited as an autosomal dominant. A coronal and a radicular variety are recognized.

Clinical Features

In the coronal variety, both deciduous and permanent dentitions are affected by abnormally formed dentin that obliterates the pulp chamber and the root canals. The enamel in the primary dentition presents a translucent, amber color. Many pulp stones are observed in the secondary dentition. In the radicular type, the tooth roots are extremely short and do not withstand occlusal forces. On that account, teeth are lost prematurely. The crown form is normal and the enamel is normal and caries-resistant. The pulp chamber is obliterated by abnormal dentin. In the molar region, the apices of the teeth are stubby and have a W-configuration. The residual pulp chamber can be made out as an inverted half-moon at the cervical margin. Premature loss of teeth is the major complication.

Differential Diagnosis (see p. 50)

Dentinogenesis imperfecta should be differentiated.

Laboratory Aids

None.

Treatment

Extraction, when indicated, with proper dental restoration is the treatment of choice.

Denture Hyperplasia (3C28)

Denture hyperplasia is a fibrous hyperplasia of the oral mucosa caused by chronic irritation due to ill-fitting dentures.

Clinical Features

Reddish pink folds of firm or flaccid fibrous connective tissue, sometimes with ulceration of intervening fissures, arise in the mucolabial and mucobuccal sulcus in contact with the flange of an ill-fitting denture. Similar folds may occur on the alveolar mucosa, especially when marked resorption of the alveolar bone has taken place. Rarely, these hyperplasias may occur over the palate under a denture or in other locations. The condition is painful only if ulceration is present. Without treatment, slow enlargement occurs.

Differential Diagnosis (see p. 37)

Squamous cell carcinoma and other soft tissue neoplasms must be considered.

Laboratory Aids

The hyperplastic tissue should be examined microscopically to rule out the possibility of squamous cell carcinoma.

Treatment

The treatment is surgical excision with construction of a new denture or relining of the old denture. Tissue conditioners are indicated.

Denture Sore Mouth (3D47)

Denture sore mouth is characterized by atrophy and inflammation of the palatal mucosa, caused by trauma and *Candida* overgrowth in the microenvironment underlying an ill-fitting denture.

Clinical Features

The mucosa beneath the upper denture is glassy, fiery red, and slightly edematous. Petechiae may be observed (3D48). The condition may be symptomless, may cause a burning sensation, or may be painful. The denture is usually unstable due to continual, prolonged use even during sleep. Untreated, the condition persists indefinitely accompanied by hyperplasia.

Differential Diagnosis (see p. 38)

Denture sore mouth is most often misdiagnosed as an allergy to denture base material. The latter is rare, but an inflammatory reaction to a component of the denture material has been reported in polymer that has not been heat-cured. Erythroplakia, a premalignant dyskeratosis in which the mucosa is also red and granular, should be considered if the condition is not strictly confined to the upper denture-bearing area.

Laboratory Aids

Candidal pseudohyphae are present but are not easily found by the methods used for acute pseudomembranous candidiasis.

Treatment

Removal and cleansing of the denture at night, sucking of topical antifungal lozenges with the denture out, and improvement of tissue tone by tissue conditioners and brushing will effect a cure. Recurrences most likely occur because the denture material harbors the fungus. In the case of recurrence, new dentures are indicated.

Dermoid Cyst (2C32)

The dermoid cyst is a developmental abnormality that occurs because of entrapment of embryonal epithelial rests within lines of embryonal fusion.

Clinical Features

Dermoid cysts can occur anywhere in the body. Those of the head and neck area do not manifest clinically until the second or third decade of life and arise most often in the floor of the mouth, either on the midline or laterally. The lesion does not have a sex predilection. When on the midline it may be located above the geniohyoid muscle, in which location it produces elevation of the tongue and occasionally compression of the epiglottis. It may also develop between the geniohyoid and the mylohyoid muscles, with occasional extension below the latter, in which case it bulges into the midline of the neck. The cyst grows very slowly. It is semisolid in consistency because it contains keratin. It varies in size, occasionally reaching large diameters.

Differential Diagnosis (see p. 23)

A great number of midline and lateral neck masses should be included, such as ranula, thyroglossal tract cyst, cystic hygroma, branchial cleft cyst, cellulitis, salivary gland pathology (either inflammatory or tumorous), and thyroid or parathyroid pathology.

Laboratory Aids

Biopsy of the lesion will reveal its cystic appearance and the presence of secondary skin appendages in the wall of the cystic mass. This will differentiate dermoid cyst from epidermoid cyst, which is essentially identical to dermoid cyst but does not contain secondary skin appendages in the cystic wall.

Treatment

Surgery is the treatment of choice.

Diphenylhydantoin Hyperplasia (3B15)

Diphenylhydantoin hyperplasia is a fibrous hyperplasia of the gingiva arising as a side effect of diphenylhydantoin therapy used in the control of epileptic convulsions and other neurologic disorders. Dental microbial plaque is central to its etiology.

Clinical Features

A diffuse enlargement of the interdental papillae and marginal gingiva is seen. The tissue is painless, nodular, firm, and pink with crevicular erythema and may become lobulated and finely pebbled. It has little tendency to bleed. The severity of the condition seems to be linked to the patient's oral hygiene and the duration of therapy. A relationship to daily dose is harder to establish. The condition starts as a marginal gingivitis followed by the enlargement of individual papillae, which may grow to cover all but the occlusal surfaces of the teeth.

Differential Diagnosis (see p. 36)

The various types of gingival fibromatosis and gingival hyperplasia associated with blood dyscrasias should be considered. Wegener's granulomatosis could also be included in the differential diagnosis.

Laboratory Aids

Biopsy reveals uniform, avascular proliferation of collagenic connective tissue almost hyaline in appearance, with overlying epithelial hyperplasia.

Treatment

Prophylaxis and excision is the indicated treatment. Surgical removal is often followed by recurrence, especially when the mouth is not kept clean. Hyperplasia is not the inevitable consequence of diphenylhydantoin therapy, for patients with good oral hygiene can avoid the condition.

Dry Socket (4E52)

Dry socket is a painful complication of tooth extraction in which a healing clot is broken down by bacteria and the bone of the tooth socket wall becomes inflamed.

Clinical Features

The tooth socket is generally empty or contains brown or broken-down blood clot fragments. The surrounding mucosa may show erythema or the trauma of a difficult extraction. Pain usually comes on 1 or 2 days after the extraction and is described as dull, boring but intense and of continuous duration. Adjacent teeth may be tender to palpation. The lymph nodes are not usually involved. A radiograph may show some degree of bone sequestration, foreign material such as calculus or dental amalgam, or tooth fragments in the socket. Resolution is usually spontaneous, fairly slow, and without complication. The commonest site of dry socket is the lower molar region. This is thought to be due to the increased thickness and relative avascularity of the mandibular bone sockets.

Differential Diagnosis (see p. 49)

The differential diagnosis should include osteitis and osteomyelitis of some other origin. Dry sockets are a frequent postextraction complication in patients with Paget's disease of bone and in patients who have undergone radiation therapy to the area.

Laboratory Aids

None.

Treatment

A variety of obtundent dressings is available. Foreign bodies should be removed from the socket.

Enamel Hypoplasia
(4A9 and 4A10; 4B20; 4B24 and 4C25)

Enamel hypoplasia is a defect in enamel formation resulting from systemic or local interference with amelogenesis. The systemic variety damages several teeth at positions on their crowns corresponding to their chronological development. The systemic causes are thought to be produced by the exanthematic diseases of childhood. The nonsystemic form presents as a localized area of hypoplasia or hypocalcification with or without hyperpigmentation (as in 4B20) and occurs on the labial aspect of the incisor teeth or on the premolar teeth adjacent to periapical infection on deciduous teeth.

Clinical Features

In the systemic form, either the deciduous or the permanent dentition is affected by a linear band of hypocalcification, pitting or hyperpigmentation. The local form (Turner's tooth) shows a labial notch (as in 4A9) that may be filled with cementum. Turner's tooth is only seen in those teeth that replace the primary dentition. Caries is always a complication in these teeth.

Differential Diagnosis (see pp. 47, 48)

Several tooth defects, such as amelogenesis imperfecta and dentinogenesis imperfecta, can be considered, especially for the systemic form.

Laboratory Aids

None.

Treatment

Large hypoplasias may need restorations.

Enamel Pearl (4A1)

Enamel pearl, or enameloma, is a local excrescence of enamel and, perhaps, dentin, rarely with dental pulp, that develops on the lateral aspect of the root surface, formed as an abnormality of root formation in which the Hertwig's root sheath assumes enamel-forming potential.

Clinical Features

Generally, enamel pearl is a symptomless, white, shiny nodule 1 or 2 mm in diameter. It is most commonly found in the bifurcation of maxillary molars. It may represent a complication only if it is involved in a periodontal pocket or if attempts are made to remove it, in which case pulp exposure could result.

Differential Diagnosis (see p. 47)

Enamel spur has a similar location and origin, the only difference being its shape. Spurs have a less bulky, triangular form.

Laboratory Aids

None.

Treatment

None.

Ephelis (1C28)

Ephelis (freckle) is a hyperpigmented macule of the skin in Caucasions that appears after exposure to sunlight. This increase in pigmentation is due to melanocytes that are more active than those in the surrounding nonaffected skin.

Clinical Features

Ephelides are generally multiple, brown, well-demarcated macules, irregularly scattered over skin that has been exposed to the sun. The oral melanotic macule is a histologically similar lesion that occasionally appears on the vermilion border of the lip or even in the oral mucosa, persisting unchanged for many years.

Differential Diagnosis (see p. 10)

Differentiation from nevus and lentigo maligna melanoma (3C36) is essentially a histologic decision. Clinically the latter tends to spread superficially, whereas ephelis remains unchanged in size.

Laboratory Aids

Biopsy should be considered to rule out lentigo maligna melanoma.

Treatment

None.

Erosion (4B15)

Erosion is a dissolution of the calcium salts of enamel and dentin produced by chemical means.

Clinical Features

Several teeth are usually affected, presenting saucer-shaped dissolution of the enamel and dentin. The site is usually related to the source of the acid, labial erosion of upper anterior teeth being associated with sucking slices of lemon or drinking acidic carbonated soft drinks. The palatal aspects of the maxillary teeth are primarily affected by acid regurgitation (pyrosis). Less commonly, the lower incisors may be affected (as in 4B15). Idiopathic erosion may also occur in various sites. Erosion is usually sufficiently slow for reactive secondary dentin to be laid down; however, if the progress of the erosion is rapid, the teeth may be extremely painful. Erosion is seen in patients with frequent episodes of vomiting and in patients with malignant neoplasms producing obstruction of the gastrointestinal tract.

Differential Diagnosis (see p. 47)

Abrasion and attrition should be differentiated, as should cervical caries. Systemic causes for frequent vomiting should be ruled out.

Laboratory Aids

None.

Treatment

The patient should be advised to avoid the source of acid.

Eruption Cyst (3A3)

Eruption cyst, or eruption hematoma, is essentially a variation of dentigerous cyst that is produced by a dilatation of the pericoronal follicular sac, creating a space above the tooth crown. This space is then occupied by serum or, most likely, blood.

Clinical Features

Eruption cyst is seen in over 90% of the cases associated with an erupting primary tooth. It has a slight predilection for females. The cyst manifests clinically as a large, red-purple bulla that covers the crown of the erupting tooth. The cyst can at times be multiple. Fluctuation is evident.

Differential Diagnosis (see p. 35)

A true dentigerous cyst as well as hemangioma and hematoma should be considered in the differential diagnosis.

Laboratory Aids

Biopsy of the lesion will demonstrate the cystic cavity, which is lined by odontogenic epithelium.

Treatment

In the great majority of cases there is no need for treatment because the erupting tooth finally will break through the cystic membrane. In some cases, however, surgical incision is indicated in order to facilitate eruption. A longitudinal incision on the surface of the cystic membrane will expose the tooth crown.

Erythema Multiforme (1B16, 1B17, and 1B18)

Erythema multiforme is a symptom complex characterized by maculopapular or vesiculobullous eruption of the skin and mucous membranes. The disorder probably is a hypersensitive reaction. Several factors, such as bacterial and viral infections, radiation therapy, and drug intake, are known to precipitate the condition, but most frequently a herpes simplex infection precedes erythema multiforme by 1 to 3 weeks.

Clinical Features

Erythema multiforme generally occurs in young adults, with a slight predilection for males. The disease has a rapid onset, and lesions may be symmetrically distributed. They are particularly common on the hands, feet, and oral mucosa. A variety of lesions may occur, usually one type predominating in a given attack. Target or iris lesions are pathognomonic when present but are frequently absent. Upper respiratory tract infection, fever, malaise, nausea, and arthralgia may occur during the early stages of the disease.

Lesions may be present anywhere on the oral mucosa. Necrotic pseudomembrane formation commonly occurs. Vesiculobullous lesions of the lips and skin rupture and become crusted. The mucous membranes of the penis, vulva, and gastrointestinal tract may be involved. Severe erythema multiforme with concomitant purulent conjunctivitis, photophobia, and leukopenia is known as the Stevens-Johnson's syndrome.

Oral lesions usually occur after skin involvement, although the sequence may be reversed in some patients. The disease is self-limiting and may last from a week to several weeks. Recurrences are common.

Secondary infection may be observed; rarely, a fulminating course may lead to a fatal outcome.

Differential Diagnosis (see p. 9)

Most vesiculobullous disorders should be considered.

Laboratory Aids

Histologic appearance is nonspecific but will rule out pemphigus vulgaris.

Treatment

There is no treatment for the condition. In severe cases corticosteroids can be used to alleviate the superimposed inflammatory symptoms.

Erythroblastosis Foetalis (4B22)

Erythroblastosis foetalis is a congenital hemolytic anemia produced by incompatibility in Rh factors of the parents. Such incompatibility occurs when the father is Rh positive (has an Rh factor) and the mother is homozygous for the Rh negative (has no Rh factor). Their newly-formed fetus will be heterozygous for the Rh factor and its positive fraction will reach the mother's circulation through the placenta. The mother's immune system will produce anti-Rh antibodies, which will induce hemolysis in the fetus. Generally, the reaction will not be evoked in the first pregnancy but only in subsequent pregnancies.

Clinical Features

The systemic manifestations, as well as oral manifestations, depend on the severity of the hemolysis. Some pregnancies with severe hemolysis result in a stillborn child. If the child is born alive, systemic manifestations will develop within the first hours or the first week after birth. These manifestations include jaundice, anemia, and generalized edema. The oral manifestations are essentially confined to the teeth. Teeth will present a typical pigmentation that varies from green to brown or various hues of blue-brown. The pigmentation is due to apposition of hemosiderin in calcified dental tissues during the period of hemolysis. Only the primary teeth are affected. Occasionally some minor degree of enamel hypoplasia can also be observed in these patients.

Differential Diagnosis (see p. 48)

Tooth pigmentations are also seen in patients under tetracycline therapy. Tetracycline fluoresces yellow under black light (or Wood light). In congenital porphyria teeth are also pigmented, but they fluoresce red under black light.

Laboratory Aids

The erythrocyte count after birth is below 1,000,000 cells per cubic millimeter.

Treatment

There is no treatment for the teeth. Only the primary teeth are affected, and the permanent dentition will not present pigmentation. The systemic treatment consists of full-body transfusion after the diagnosis is rendered.

Fibroepithelial Polyp (2C27; 2D43; 3E55)

Fibroepithelial polyp is a nonneoplastic overgrowth of fibrous connective tissue of traumatic origin.

Clinical Features

The lesion is usually found on the buccal mucosa opposite the occlusal plane of the teeth as a firm or slightly compressible polypoid mass (as in 2C27). Other trauma-prone sites, such as the lateral border and tip of the tongue (as in 2D43), the lips, and the palate (as in 3E55), can be the site of this lesion. The growth arrests as the lesion matures, and it is generally covered by a layer of keratin. Therefore, it is white.

Differential Diagnosis (see pp. 23, 24, 38)

Several conditions such as a true fibroma, neurofibroma, and neurilemoma, among others, should be considered in the differential diagnosis. Peripheral giant cell granuloma and pyogenic granuloma can be excluded because they are well vascularized. Therefore, their color is markedly different. Papillomas or condyloma accuminatum (venereal warts) present a cauliflowerlike surface. If the lesion

is multiple, neurofibromatosis of von Recklinghausen and other neurocrestopath-
ies should be considered.

Laboratory Aids

Biopsy of the lesion will reveal a mass of mature fibrous connective tissue
covered by a hyperplastic and hyperkeratinized epithelium.

Treatment

Surgical excision is the treatment of choice.

Fibrosarcoma (3C27)

Fibrosarcoma is a malignant neoplasm of fibrous connective tissue that can also arise in bone.

Clinical Features

Fibrosarcoma is rare in the head and neck region. Intraorally, it can occur anywhere. It generally affects the sexes equally, with the highest incidence in patients
between 20 and 40 years of age. Cases in infants and young children are known
to occur. Fibrosarcoma does not have a marked tendency to metastasize.

The lesion presents with uncontrolled growth (either rapid or slow), mobility
of teeth, and bone destruction. It is generally a painless, sessile swelling that may
ulcerate. Pain arises with involvement of nerve terminals.

Differential Diagnosis (see p. 37)

Any intraoral growth showing malignant characteristics could be included in
the differential diagnosis. A spectrum of low-grade fibrosarcomas with a relatively
benign course (dermatofibroma protuberans), difficult to differentiate from reactive fibroses of various kinds (desmoid tumor), has been rarely reported in oral
soft tissues.

Laboratory Aids

Biopsy will show the nature of the lesion.

Treatment

Radical surgery is the treatment of choice. Radiation therapy seems to have
no effect on this neoplasm.

Fibrous Dysplasia of Bone, Monostotic
(5A9 and 5A10; 5C31)

Monostotic fibrous dysplasia is a dysplastic process of bone that is not well understood. The condition is of unknown etiology. Some investigators claim a traumatic and/or inflammatory etiology, but this is not fully sustained.

Clinical Features

Monostotic fibrous dysplasia can affect any bone in the body. The maxilla and mandible are among the frequently affected bones. The condition does not have a sex predilection. It is most frequently seen in children and young adults. In either the maxilla or the mandible it begins as a painless enlargement. In the mandible it expands both lingual and buccal plates. In the maxilla it tends to arise in the tuberosity, and, therefore, it expands into the maxillary sinus or into the palate. Erasure of the vestibular sulcus is also seen, but the mucosa overlying the enlargement is within normal limits. The process is not encapsulated and, therefore, poses a serious problem for treatment. Especially difficult are those cases that develop in the maxilla, which, after extending into the maxillary sinus, progressively displace the orbital floor. The growth is expansile, and the lesion may become tender in later stages. Variation in size is well known. Both minute lesions of a few centimeters and grotesque facial deformities have been observed. Nevertheless, the condition is self-limiting, and when it begins in childhood it generally stops growing at puberty. The process never produces paresthesia or resorption of tooth roots.

Various radiographic appearances can be seen. There is a cystic variety in which a radiolucency of variable size can be observed with occasional spicules of bone formation and a well-circumscribed periphery. Sometimes this type shows a radiolucency with a marked degree of bone trabeculation traversing the lesion. Other cases may show frank bone formation demonstrating the so-called ground glass appearance or orange peel appearance on roentgenograms.

Differential Diagnosis (see pp. 59, 60)

Depending on the location, the differential diagnosis includes a great number of conditions, such as periapical pathology, traumatic bone cyst, osteoid osteoma, ossifying fibroma, odontogenic tumor, and central giant cell lesion of bone. The final diagnosis is achieved by careful interrogation of the patient, clinical examination, good radiographs, and biopsy.

Laboratory Aids

Biopsy will indicate the nature of the lesion. Histologically, the differential diagnosis should be established between monostotic and polystotic varieties with lesions such as ossifying fibroma of bone, benign osteoblastoma and other so-called fibroosseous lesions of bone.

Treatment

It is difficult in some cases, especially in the jaws and most particularly in the maxilla, to fully excise this lesion, because it does not have definite borders. The treatment of choice is surgery, and, when complete excision is not possible, the patient is treated by conservative removal of the portion of the lesion that accentuates the facial malformation. Repeated surgical procedures are undertaken when needed. These lesions should never be treated with radiation therapy, since it is well-known that they will undergo malignant transformation into an osteogenic sarcoma.

Fibrous Dysplasia of Bone, Polyostotic
(5A7 and 5A8)

Polyostotic fibrous dysplasia is characterized by multiple radiolucent bone lesions of unknown etiology. In addition, the majority of affected females and some affected males present precocious puberty.

Clinical Features

Two varieties of polyostotic fibrous dysplasia should be distinguished. One is the so-called Albright's syndrome, which is characterized by multiple, bony lesions and precocious puberty in the female. The other variety is called Jaffe's type of polyostotic fibrous dysplasia, in which the bone lesions are similar to those in Albright's variety but precocious puberty is not present. Any bone in the body can be affected and the degree of involvement can range from very mild to very severe, demonstrating large radiolucencies. The presence of lesions on the legs will produce bowing of the femur. These lesions can be asymptomatic, or they can present with marked pain. Fracture is a frequent complication, especially in the large bones. When lesions develop in the facial skeleton they are hypertrophic, resulting in facial asymmetry, and if they are present in the maxilla they may even induce exophthalmus and obliteration of the maxillary sinuses. Maxillary lesions very frequently present a ground-glass appearance on radiographic examination. Displacement of teeth can also be observed in large lesions. Systemic manifestations include pigmentation of the skin, described as café-au-lait type. This pigmentation is scattered over different areas, especially the forehead and buttocks; occasionally pigmentation of the lips and oral mucosa has been observed. Females are affected with precocious puberty, and generally the first menses begins at anywhere from 1 to 5 years of age. Males occasionally develop precocious puberty with capability of fertilization.

Differential Diagnosis (see p. 59)

The differential diagnosis of the polyostotic type of fibrous dysplasia should include a large number of conditions, such as histiocytosis X, parathyroidism, and neurofibromatosis, among others.

Laboratory Aids

In about one-half of the patients, alkyline phosphatase levels in serum have been found to be elevated. Biopsy of one of the lesions will demonstrate its nature.

Treatment

Unfortunately, this condition tends to be spread throughout different bones of the body, making surgical treatment impossible. Some individuals have attempted radiation therapy, but this is a very dangerous procedure, for these lesions, after radiation, tend to undergo transformation into osteogenic sarcoma. Single or very well delineated lesions can be treated with surgical procedures.

Fibrous Gingival Hyperplasia (3C30)

Fibrous gingival hyperplasia is an overgrowth of gingival fibrous connective tissue, sometimes forming amorphous calcification or bone. It is caused by minor trauma or mechanical or microbial irritation.

Clinical Features

Clinically, this condition is generally a pale pink, or red and pink, sessile or pedunculate mass or masses of at most 1 cm in diameter usually present on the interdental marginal gingiva. Its consistency may vary with the fibrous or bony content. Slow growth arrests with maturation.

Differential Diagnosis (see p. 37)

Pyogenic granuloma, peripheral giant cell granuloma, and gingival cyst or neoplasia should be considered.

Laboratory Aids

Biopsy will demonstrate the nature of the lesion.

Treatment

Surgical excision is the treatment of choice.

Fissured Tongue (2E51)

Fissured or scrotal tongue is of unknown etiology. Recent evidence seems to indicate a multifactorial etiology.

Clinical Features

The fissures are multiple and symmetrically disposed, either around a deep central fissure or on the lateral aspect of the tongue, and they seem to increase with age. They vary considerably in number, size, and depth. The condition is asymptomatic, unless complicated by geographic tongue or candidiasis (as in 2E51). Fissured tongue can be found in association with acromegaly, Down's syndrome, Melkersson-Rosenthal's syndrome, and Sjögren's syndrome.

Differential Diagnosis (see p. 25)

The clinical appearance is so typical that the final diagnosis is self-evident.

Laboratory Aids

None.

Treatment

Brushing of the tongue is indicated, as is treatment with antifungal agents if the condition is secondarily infected with *Candida.*

Florid Osseous Dysplasia (5C26)

Florid osseous dysplasia, which has been described under a great variety of names, is an abnormality of the tooth-bearing area of the maxilla and mandible in which large, densely calcified masses resembling cementum are deposited in the periodontium and neighboring alveolar bone. This lesion may also be accompanied by solitary bone cysts.

Clinical Features

Lesions generally occur simultaneously in all four quadrants of the jaws. Radiographically they present mostly as a diffuse radiopacity with a cotton wool appearance similar to that seen in Paget's disease of bone. These radiopacities may be associated with areas of radiolucency, observed both in the alveolar bone and in the periodontium. The non-tooth-bearing areas of both jaws are not affected by the process. The condition appears to have a predilection for black women; however, cases have been reported in both sexes and in other races. The lesions are not well circumscribed, and there may be gross expansion of the cortical plates resembling fibrous dysplasia or Paget's disease. Their behavior is one of very gradual expansion over a number of years without pain. The changes are generally discovered on routine roentgenographic examination. The resistance of the bone to infection may be impaired and osteomyelitis may supervene.

Differential Diagnosis (see p. 60)

The expansion of bone and apparent hypercementosis may simulate Paget's disease of bone. A condition known as dominant familial cemental dysplasia has a similar radiologic appearance, but it has been observed in several kindreds.

Certain features of florid osseous dysplasia and dominant familial cemental dysplasia are similar enough that these two entities still need further classification.

Laboratory Aids

Serum calcium, phosphorus, and alkaline phosphatase appear to be within normal limits.

Treatment

It is probable that the treatment should be confined to cosmetic surgery and diagnostic biopsy. Rigorous dental hygiene and regular dental checkups are required to avoid the complications of dental infection.

Fluorosis, Dental (4B21)

The effect of excess fluoride on the teeth is manifested as white or brown patches that produce a mottled appearance. Enamel mottling due to fluoride intake is geographical in distribution, being observed in parts of the world where the water naturally contains high levels of fluoride.

Clinical Features

The teeth affected are those exposed to high levels of dietary fluoride. Variable degrees of involvement are observed. Mottling is generally scattered over the teeth. The perikymata may be accentuated by alternating light and dark bands, and in severe cases pitting and lack of tissue may be present, resulting in loss of normal tooth form. The primary dentition is generally less affected than the permanent dentition. Fluorosis will tend to occur when the concentration of fluoride in the water is greater than 2 parts per million. Higher levels will be accompanied by systemic fluorosis with bone changes such as osteosclerosis and renal and abdominal problems. Dental changes depend not only on fluoride concentration but also on unknown individual variances.

Differential Diagnosis (see p. 48)

Severe cases should be differentiated from amelogenesis imperfecta. Advanced cases of tetracycline intake could also be considered.

Laboratory Aids

None.

Treatment

Advanced cases require restorative dental procedures.

Fordyce's Granules (2C25)

Fordyce's granules are a variant of normal mucosa in which heterotopic sebaceous glands are present.

Clinical Features

Bilateral, symptomless, brownish yellow, sebaceous glands are seen in the superficial lamina propria. They are usually found in the buccal mucosa or in the inner surface of the lips and less commonly in other oral sites such as the soft palate. They are present in about 80% of the adult population, apparently increasing in number at puberty. Rarely, an intraoral sebaceous adenoma may occur. (Also illustrated in 2B25 are petechial hemorrhages of the vestibule secondary to operative procedures.)

Differential Diagnosis (see p. 23)

The clinical appearance is so typical that the final diagnosis is self-evident.

Laboratory Aids

None, but if a biopsy is performed, the typical normal-looking sebaceous glands will be observed.

Treatment

None.

Foreign Body (2A2; 2A3 and 2A4)

Foreign bodies implanted in the oral soft tissues, if inert, may provoke no local response. If they are not inert, fibrosis, chronic inflammation, formation of abscess, and discharge from a sinus (as in 2A2) may occur.

Clinical Features

The foreign body is usually not visible but is frequently palpable. However, with excess scarring, the contours may not be perceived very well. (In 2A3 a gold radon implant shines through the labial mucosa.) The foreign body, if sufficiently radiopaque, is demonstrable by radiograph (as in 2A4). Therefore, the soft tissues of the lip in children who have fractured anterior teeth should be radiographed. Complications are generally confined to scarring and infection around the inflammatory focus.

Differential Diagnosis (see p. 21)

Depending on the location, certain lesions such as sialolith and epidermoid cyst should be considered.

Laboratory Aids

None.

Treatment

Surgical removal of the foreign body is indicated.

Fracture, Bone (5D47; 5D48 and 5E49)

Fractures of the maxilla and mandible may be either traumatic or pathologic, the most common cause being an accident or a blow to the area.

Clinical Features

Traumatic fractures of the head and neck area occur at the following sites (in order of frequency): the neck of the condylar process of the ramus of the mandible, the angle of the mandible, the body of the mandible, and the premolar region. Horizontal alveolar fractures (as in 5E49) are relatively uncommon. In the maxilla the anterior segment is most frequently involved. Pathological fractures occur in association with large cysts and neoplasms. Fractures present clinically with disordered occlusion, occasionally with trismus, ecchymosis in the floor of the mouth, and mobility and/or fracture of the teeth. External lacerations (as in 5E48) may be present. Dental complications may be loss of tooth vitality and root resorption (as in 5E49). Infection of the bone through poorly immobilized bone fragments, particularly with a tooth in the line of fracture, may result in osteomyelitis.

Differential Diagnosis (see pp. 61, 62)

Radiographs will demonstrate the fracture, making the diagnosis self-evident.

Laboratory Aids

None.

Treatment

Intradental wiring, splinting, and transosseous wiring may be required. Antibiotics for the control of infection should be considered in complex fractures. Teeth in the line of fracture should be removed.

Fracture, Tooth (4A2)

Fractures of the enamel and dentin, with exposure of the tooth pulp, are most common in childhood as a result of a great variety of traumas, the most common being a fall against an object or a blow from contact with another child or from a flying object.

Clinical Features

The most commonly injured teeth are the maxillary central incisors, followed by the maxillary lateral incisors, with no significant difference between the sexes. The presentation depends on the depth and the direction of the fracture. Superficial fractures of the enamel and the dentin present as a rough, ragged chipping that is generally painless (though there may be some sensitivity). Deeper fractures, involving more dentin, expose numerous dentinal tubules and are painful. These horizontal fractures are subject to infection through the open tubules. The pulp may be seen to shine through as a pink mass. If the pulp is exposed, bleeding may occur. In contrast to horizontal or oblique fractures, vertical fractures involving enamel, dentin, and pulp and obliquely involving the root with retention of both fragments may provide a difficult diagnostic test. The use of a sharp explorer and dental disclosing solution may be helpful to delineate the fracture line. Superficial fractures of enamel and dentin have good prognosis; however, deeper fractures in dentin have a tendency to allow infection to extend to the pulp. A simultaneous contusion of the apical blood vessels causes loss of pulp vitality.

Differential Diagnosis (see p. 47)

The clinical appearance is so evident as not to warrant a differential diagnosis.

Laboratory Aids

Radiographs and tooth vitality tests must always be done on initial presentation.

Treatment

Treatment is dependent on the involvement of the dentin and pulp and the mobility of the fragments and may involve pulp capping, pulp extirpation, splinting, and root canal therapy.

Gardner's Syndrome (5A6)

Gardner's syndrome is characterized by multiple osteomas, especially of the facies; epidermoid inclusion cysts of the skin, which may be present in the face, trunk, and extremities, usually appearing after puberty; polyposis of the large intestine that eventually undergoes malignant transformation; and fibromas and desmoid tumors of the skin or mesentery or both, as well as lipomas or lipofibromas or both. The condition is inherited in an autosomal dominant manner with variable expressivity and marked penetrance.

Clinical Features

Multiple osteomas may be found in the calvaria and facial skeleton. The frontal bone is the most frequent site of occurrence of the osteomas, and they generally precede the appearance of the intestinal polyposis. The osteomas expand and ob-literate the paranasal sinuses, especially the sphenoid and ethmoid sinuses.

Osteomas are also frequent in the maxilla and mandible. In more than half of the reported cases, compound odontomas have been described as part of the syndrome, as have hypercementosis and unerupted teeth.

Multiple intestinal polyposis of the colon and rectum with a marked tendency to malignant degeneration is the most serious component of this syndrome. The polyps may appear before puberty.

Fibromas and desmoid tumors of the skin and mesentery, as well as lipomas, may also be present. Epidermoid inclusion cysts of the skin generally appear after puberty. Osteomas may also occur in long bones.

Differential Diagnosis (see p. 59)

Intestinal polyposis of types I, II, and IV, juvenile-type polyposis coli, and multiple hamartoma syndrome should be included in the differential diagnosis.

Laboratory Aids

Roentgenographic examination of the skeleton and barium contrast survey of the large and small bowel are suggested.

Treatment

Orally, odontomas are surgically excised, as are small osteomas of the jaws. Preventive surgery of the colonic polyposis is indicated in order to avoid malignant transformation. Proper genetic counseling is imperative for this syndrome.

Garré's Osteitis (5E53)

Garré's osteitis (chronic osteomyelitis with proliferative periosteitis) is an excess of subperiosteal bone formed in response to a chronic inflammatory stimulus. It is located centrally in the bone, usually the mandible and it is related to a pericoronal or periapical infection.

Clinical Features

This condition manifests as a single fusiform swelling approximately 3 cm long found on the buccal aspect or lower border of the mandible, most commonly adjacent to the source of infection. Pain, especially on chewing, may emanate from the site of infection. The swelling is hard and on a radiograph appears as an elevation of the periosteum with subperiosteal bone formation, which may be lamellated, presenting an onionskin appearance. The condition generally resolves after removal of the septic focus.

Differential Diagnosis (see p. 62)

Radiographically the onionskin appearance can be seen in other entities, such as Ewing's sarcoma. Careful interrogation of the patient, clinical inspection, and radiographic survey will demonstrate the precise nature of the lesion.

Laboratory Aids

None.

Treatment

Treatment is extraction of the tooth, after which the bony mass will diminish in size.

Gemination (4A7 and 4A8)

Traditionally, gemination is defined as a subtype of fusion in which the fused teeth are formed by the union of two supernumerary teeth or by the union of one supernumerary tooth with a regular tooth. (Fusion is the union between any two teeth.) There is a great variation in the accepted definitions for these entities.

Clinical Features

Clinically, both gemination and fusion manifest as two teeth fused together, occasionally with partial degrees of separation, especially at the level of the incisal edge. The most frequent teeth involved in either gemination or fusion are the anterior maxillary teeth and the mandibular incisor. There is a significant sex predilection, males being affected twice as frequently as females.

Differential Diagnosis (see p. 47)

Gemination and fusion of teeth are very difficult to distinguish from one another; however, both are readily differentiated from other conditions.

Laboratory Aids

Radiographs will show two teeth fused together.

Treatment

Treatment generally consists of aesthetic repair of the area, if possible, or construction of a prosthesis.

Giant Cell Granuloma, Central (5E52)

The central giant cell granuloma of the jaw is a nonneoplastic condition of unknown etiology. This lesion is probably closely related to the aneurysmal bone cyst. In fact, these two lesions have been reported arising together in the same patient. Several theories have been proposed to explain the etiology, including neoplasia and trauma. It is worthwhile to note that central giant cell granuloma occurs only in the jaws and is unknown in other bones of the body.

Clinical Features

The condition has a predilection for females, affecting from 2 to 5 females (depending on the statistic) for every male. The majority of the cases occur in the molar-premolar mandibular body area in patients generally less than 15 years of age. Cases in the maxilla have also been described. Central giant cell granuloma has an expansile growth but does not destroy the cortical plate and as a rule is asymptomatic. When it reaches a large size, it produces facial asymmetry. Radiographically it is characterized by a large area of radiolucency that may be transversed by very delicate bony spicules. When the lesion occurs in the mandibular symphysis, it will tend to cross the midline. Displacement of teeth may be apparent in larger lesions.

Differential Diagnosis (see p. 62)

The differential diagnosis can include a great variety of odontogenic and bone tumors, but those that must be considered are monostotic fibrous dysplasia, traumatic bone cyst, and aneurysmal bone cyst.

Laboratory Aids

Biopsy of the lesion will demonstrate a mature connective tissue stroma with large numbers of multinucleated giant cells of the osteoclastic type.

Treatment

The treatment of choice is surgical excision.

Giant Cell Granuloma, Peripheral (3C32)

Peripheral giant cell granuloma is most likely a reactive response to trauma or some inflammatory process. The lesion occurs on the mucosal surfaces and generally has a deep area of implantation.

Clinical Features

This granuloma varies in appearance according to the site. The lesion can be sessile or pedunculated. It is frequently located in the gingiva or alveolar mucosa. It presents as an exophytic mass with a purple-brown color because of its high vascularity. The lesions range in size from very small to more than 2 cm in diameter. They can be found at any age but are most likely seen in patients over 30 years of age. Radiographically there is generally no evidence of bone involvement, but in some cases one can see a slight superficial bone erosion.

Differential Diagnosis (see p. 37)

Pyogenic granuloma and pregnancy tumor should be included in the differential diagnosis. Rarely will any other lesions of the gingiva present with this type of clinical appearance.

Laboratory Aids

Biopsy of the lesion will reveal the presence of large numbers of multinucleated giant cells of the osteoclastic type. In addition, one can observe a very well vascularized connective tissue stroma and occasional areas of dystrophic calcification.

Treatment

The treatment is surgical excision, and care must be taken to eliminate the base of the lesion. If the attachment to either bone or periodontal ligament is not properly eliminated, the lesion will tend to recur.

Gingival Cyst of the Adult (4E53 and 4E54)

This cyst occurs entirely within soft gingival tissue, and its etiology is believed to be either cystic degeneration of rests of the dental lamina or traumatic implantation of surface epithelium.

Clinical Features

In the great majority of cases, this lesion occurs at the level of the mandibular cuspid and/or bicuspid, most in individuals over 40 years of age. There is generally a well-circumscribed elevation of the gingiva, normal in color and not exceeding 1 cm in greatest dimension. This soft tissue lesion may occasionally produce superficial erosion of the alveolar bone. Some authors consider this entity a superficial location of the lateral periodontal cyst. However, the distinction should be made between the two entities because of probable different etiology and slightly different treatment necessitated by the fact that the gingival cyst is very superficially located whereas the lateral periodontal cyst is entirely within bone.

Differential Diagnosis (see p. 50)

This entity could be confused with a mucocele. The differential diagnosis could also include some other neoplastic pathology of the gingiva as well as inflammatory processes of periodontal origin (i.e., abscess).

Laboratory Aids

None.

Treatment

Conservative surgical excision is the treatment of choice.

Gingival Cyst of the Newborn (3A2)

Gingival cyst of the newborn is also known as dental lamina cyst of the newborn, Epstein's pearls, or Bohn's nodules. The etiology of this entity is considered a cystic degeneration of epithelial rests from the dental lamina.

Clinical Features

The condition is present at birth and is generally observed in either the maxillary or mandibular buccal gingiva, or both. It is characterized by multiple white nodules of various sizes distributed throughout the aforementioned areas and occasionally on the hard palate. In the majority of cases, the cysts are confined to very minute swellings, but occasionally they can be so large as to be clinically obvious. They seem to be asymptomatic.

Differential Diagnosis (see p. 35)

This condition is so unique as to have almost no differential diagnosis. Nevertheless, congenital bony exostosis should be considered.

Laboratory Aids

None.

Treatment

These cysts generally need no treatment. Within a few days they open spontaneously and disappear. A large cyst that does not disappear within a week after birth can be surgically curetted.

Gingival Fibromatosis (3B16)

There are several forms of gingival fibromatoses characterized by a generalized enlargement of the gingiva. Some are idiopathic, whereas others are hereditary or inflammatory in nature. The hereditary variants identified here are extremely rare.

Clinical Features

All of the forms of gingival fibromatosis identified here share their oral appearance as a diffuse enlargement of the gingiva that generally coincides with the eruption of the primary incisors. This soft tissue proliferation is noninflammatory and it appears normal in color and texture. This hypertrophic growth is progressive and eventually covers the crown of the tooth.

Lingual fibromatosis with hypertrichosis is characterized by epilepsy, mental retardation, and hypertrichosis in addition to gingival fibromatosis. The mental retardation and epilepsy are inconsistent features. The syndrome is inherited in an autosomal dominant manner. The facies is characterized by protrusion of the lips, secondary to gingival enlargement, and hypertrichosis, especially of the eyebrows.

Gingival fibromatosis with ear, nose, bone, and nail defects is characterized by dysplasia of nails; soft, bulky cartilage in the nose and ears; hepatosplenomegaly; and hypoplastic terminal phalanges. The condition is inherited in an autosomal dominant manner.

Gingival fibromatosis with multiple hyaline fibromas is characterized by hypertrophy of the gingiva; hypertrophy of the nail beds; and fibrotic tumors of the nose, chin, head, and palmar and digital surfaces of the hands. The condition is inherited in an autosomal recessive manner. Fibrotic hyaline tumors appear on the nose, chin, and head usually after the age of 2. Multiple fibrous tumors resembling those on the face appear on the back, fingers, thighs, and legs, often producing flexion contractures at the knees, elbows, shoulders, and hips.

Differential Diagnosis (see p. 36)

Isolated gingival fibromatosis and gingival fibromatosis secondary to *Dilantin* therapy (3B15) should be considered in establishing the diagnosis. In the case of multiple hyaline fibromas, neurofibromatosis, Gardner's syndrome, and fibromatosis hyalinica multiplex juvenilis, should be considered. Buccal exostosis associated with gingival hyperplasia (3B16) should also be considered in the differential diagnosis.

Laboratory Aids

None.

Treatment

Surgical correction can be attempted, but the condition is known to recur. In those cases in which teeth have been extracted, the gingiva resumes its normal position.

Gingivitis, Chronic Marginal, and Periodontitis
(3B20; 3B21 and 3B22; 4B18)

Chronic marginal gingivitis is a destructive inflammation thought to be due to the diffusion of toxic products or antigens from bacterial plaque through the gingival crevicular epithelium. No one organism has been found to be the cause. Inflammatory cells and fluid exudate derived from the serum emerge from the gingival crevice.

Clinical Features

The marginal gingiva becomes red and slightly swollen. Chronic marginal gingivitis and periodontitis are generally painless; however, a dull ache may be felt, particularly after meals, and is subjectively felt to be relieved by sucking the teeth (as in 3B20). Gingival bleeding after meals or toothbrushing is a frequent symptom of gingivitis. Loosening of the teeth may bring the patient to the dentist at a relatively late stage, for if not arrested as gingivitis the condition progresses to chronic periodontitis, in which periodontal pockets are formed between the epithelium and connective tissue of the gingiva and the cementum of the tooth. This is accompanied by destruction of the collagen fibers of the periodontal ligament and resorption of the alveolar bone. These pockets provide a microenvironment favorable to the development of further dental plaque, which may calcify to form calculus, and pockets tend to migrate apically on the tooth, making the tooth mobile (as in 3B21 and 3B22). On occasion, bacteria may infect the alveolar bone and provoke the formation of a periodontal abscess.

Differential Diagnosis (see pp. 36, 47)

The differential diagnosis should include gingivitis of various origins.

Laboratory Aids

Plaque indices and measurements of fluid from the gingival crevice correlate with the severity of the disease.

Treatment

Gingivitis and to an extent periodontitis are reversible and preventable by good oral hygiene, provided no adverse local or systemic factors interfering with healing are present in the patient. Periodontal surgery is aimed at eliminating pockets and gaining reattachment of the gingiva to healthy tooth substance.

Globulomaxillary Cyst (5E58)

Globulomaxillary cyst was once thought to be of developmental origin based upon the idea that it develops from epithelial rests trapped in the line of fusion between the globular process and the maxillary process. Today, this theory is not very well accepted. Recent evidence points to the fact that this entity probably represents an odontogenic keratocyst in this particular location.

Clinical Features

The cyst occurs, as classically described, between the lateral incisor and the maxillary cuspid teeth. There is no clinical symptomatology. Pulp vitality is within normal limits for these two teeth. The majority of the cysts have been discovered on routine radiographic examination. Radiographically the lesion has a typical inverted pear shape.

Examples have been seen in which the cyst has induced divergence of the roots of the neighboring teeth.

Differential Diagnosis (see p. 62)

The differential diagnosis should include an unusual lateral periodontal cyst and an apical cyst associated with either the lateral incisor or the cuspid tooth in the area. Pulp vitality of both lateral incisor and canine teeth should always be tested. Neoplastic bone pathology also should be ruled out.

Laboratory Aids

None.

Treatment

The treatment of choice is surgery. The adjacent teeth should be preserved since they are vital.

Granular Cell Myoblastoma (2D42)

Granular cell myoblastoma is an uncommon benign neoplasm of debatable origin. Some theories propose an origin in striated muscle, but tumors have been found in areas in which striated muscle does not normally develop. Other cells, such as histiocytes and neural crest cells, have been implicated as sites of origin.

Clinical Features

Granular cell myoblastoma in the oral cavity most likely develops in the body of the tongue. The neoplasm is usually a single node, generally protruding on the ventral surface of the tongue, with a yellowish color. It has no sex and/or age predilection. Granular cell myoblastoma grows very slowly and is painless.

Differential Diagnosis (see p. 24)

The differential diagnosis should include a variety of lesions that could occur in the tongue, such as fibroma, inflammatory hyperplasia, neurilemoma, and neurofibroma among the most frequent. Final diagnosis can be established after microscopic examination.

Laboratory Aids

Biopsy will demonstrate the nature of the lesion.

Treatment

The treatment is surgical excision. The neoplasm does not tend to recur if properly treated.

Hairy Tongue (2E57)

Hairy tongue is an elongation of the filiform papillae, which become pigmented to varying degrees by chromogenic bacteria, fungi, or tobacco. The condition is frequently secondary to antibiotic therapy and is harmless.

Clinical Features

The dorsum of the tongue is symmetrically covered by a thick coat of enlarged hyperkeratinized filiform papillae resembling hairs. These may be black, brown, or yellow; hence the different names used (e.g., black hairy tongue). No nodes are palpable.

The condition is usually accidentally discovered. It persists for days and even weeks and disappears spontaneously. The only complication may be occasional gagging.

Differential Diagnosis (see p. 25)

Pigmentation of the tongue due to fruits, candy, drugs containing bismuth, and decomposed blood lying between the papillae may also simulate this condition.

Laboratory Aids

None.

Treatment

Brushing the tongue should be tried, but if the condition persists topical triamcinolone acetonide (*Kenalog*) or nystatin suspension should be used. The condition is not a contraindication to an essential antibiotic regimen, but it should be anticipated when the antibiotic is reused at a later date.

Hand-Foot-and-Mouth Disease (2E59)

Hand-foot-and-mouth disease is an acute viral infection characterized by vesicle formation on both the skin and the oral mucosa. The condition is epidemic in nature and is caused by various Coxsackie viruses, especially group B, type 16. This disorder is in no way related to the so-called hoof-and-mouth disease of cattle.

Clinical Features

The disorder almost invariably occurs in children between 1 and 10 years of age, with a peak incidence between 1 and 5 years. Adults are seldom affected. The virus has an estimated incubation period of from 2 to 6 days. A subfebrile stage and mild malaise are characteristic. The initial lesions are red papules, 2 to 10 mm in diameter. Within 2 days, the papules become grayish vesicles scattered over the sides of the palms and soles and on the ventral surfaces of the fingers and toes. They range from 20 to 100 in number. Oral lesions are similar to skin lesions, but they are fewer in number (ranging from 5 to 10) and their vesicular stage is shorter. After rupture, painful aphthouslike lesions are seen, especially on the lips and buccal mucosa. Regional lymphadenitis is rare.

The condition is self-limiting and lasts anywhere from 1 to 2 weeks. There are no known complications. Hand-foot-and-mouth disease is highly contagious. Therefore, extra care in handling these patients is necessary.

Differential Diagnosis (see p. 25)

The typical lesions of the oral cavity, hands, and feet should exclude almost all other vesicular and ulcerative conditions.

Laboratory Aids

Complement fixation and inoculation of guinea pigs or suckling mice are used for diagnosis of the disease and isolation of the virus. Intracytoplasmic viral inclusion bodies can occasionally be identified in cells obtained from scraping of the lesions.

Treatment

A topical anesthetic can be used to control pain in the oral lesions.

Hemangioma (1E54; 2A12; 2D45)

Hemangioma is a benign neoplasm of vascular tissue characterized by proliferation of numerous small capillaries or large, endothelial-lined, cavernous spaces. The so-called flat hemangiomas observed on the skin (birthmarks) and occasionally in the oral cavity are congenital and considered to be a developmental anomaly rather than a neoplasm.

Clinical Features

Intraoral hemangiomas can occur in almost any area of the oral mucosa and occasionally within bone. The most frequent sites are the tongue, the lip and the buccal mucosa. Clinically the lesion can be either flat or exophytic and occasionally is multilobulated. Its color is deep purple, in contrast to hematoma, which has a dark brown color. Hemangiomas are asymptomatic and in the great majority of cases are present from birth. Once they reach a certain size, they tend to remain stationary. Occasionally, mastication or other trauma may produce superficial ulcerations with bleeding episodes. Hemangiomas are generally not well demarcated from the neighboring tissues. When an intrabony lesion occurs, it will most likely be located in the body of the mandible, presenting a radiolucent, honeycomb appearance on X ray. It is recommended that, whenever this type of radiolucency shows up in the mandible, an aspiration biopsy be contemplated in order to rule out the possibility of intrabony hemangioma. Surgical opening of this type of lesion can result in severe hemorrhage.

Differential Diagnosis (see pp. 12, 22, 24)

If the lesion is observed in the soft tissue, hematoma, lymphangioma, and hemangiomas associated with Sturge-Weber's syndrome should be considered. One must remember that malignant tumors of capillary formation, such as hemangio-endothelioma and angiosarcoma, do exist and should be included in the differential diagnosis.

Laboratory Aids

Biopsy of the lesion will reveal the numerous capillaries, as described.

Treatment

A great number of congenital hemangiomas generally undergo regression toward puberty. Cases that do not regress or cases present in older individuals can be treated by a variety of means, including surgery or, better, a combination of sclerosing agents and surgery. As mentioned, caution during surgery is imperative in order to avoid severe hemorrhage.

Hematoma (2B13; 2D44; 3D39 and 3D40)

Hematoma, or blood blister, is a traumatic extravasation of blood into tissue spaces.

Clinical Features

A subepithelial, bluish red macule or vesicle that can be related to a site of trauma is commonly found opposite the occlusal plane of the teeth. Some deep hematomas arise as a result of trauma to vessels during administration of local anesthetics. The lesion tends to become yellowish brown and fades within two weeks.

Differential Diagnosis (see pp. 22, 24, 37)

Petechial hemorrhages, large hematomas, and ecchymoses occur intraorally in the bleeding diatheses.

Laboratory Aids

None.

Treatment

In recurrent cases due to self-biting the patient should be instructed to abandon the habit.

Hereditary Hemorrhagic Telangiectasia (1C30)

Hereditary hemorrhagic telangiectasia is characterized by multiple capillary and venous dilations of the skin and mucous membranes with recurrent episodes of hemorrhage. The condition is inherited as an autosomal dominant. Time of onset is usually during the second or third decade.

Clinical Features

Pinpoint, spiderlike telangiectases are observed on the face, nasal orifices, ears, scalp, eyelids, and lips. Lesions on the nasal mucosa produce frequent and occasionally severe epistaxis that may persist for several days. Nosebleed generally precedes the appearance of cutaneous lesions.

Telangiectases affect the lip and its mucocutaneous junction, the anterior dorsum and tip of the tongue, and occasionally the palate, the gingiva, and the buccal mucosa. Bleeding from the oral cavity, especially from the lips and tongue, succeeds epistaxis.

Mucous membranes in the gastrointestinal tract, conjunctiva, vagina, and any organ (e.g., brain, spinal cord, lungs, liver) may be affected with telangiectases that hemorrhage.

Differential Diagnosis (see p. 10)

The syndrome should be differentiated from angiokeratoma corporis diffusum (Fabry's syndrome), and CRST (calcinosis, Raynaud's phenomenon, sclerodactyly, and telangiectasia) syndrome.

Laboratory Aids

None.

Treatment

Treatment consists of controlling hemorrhagic episodes by different homeostatic means. In cases requiring intraoral operative procedures, caution should be exercised so as not to accidentally injure neighboring tissues.

Hereditary Opalescent Dentin (4B23; 4C34)

Hereditary opalescent dentin, also known as dentinogenesis imperfecta, is a developmental disturbance of dentin inherited as an autosomal dominant.

Clinical Features

Both deciduous and permanent dentitions are affected by hypoplasia of dentin, resulting in a bluish brown, amberlike hue to the teeth. The overlying enamel has a tendency to chip and to become readily eroded, and caries may supervene. Crown form, in the posterior area, has a tendency to be bulbous, and roots are short and conical (as in 4C34). The pulp chambers and root canals are obliterated. Attrition of the tooth crowns is rapid. By way of complication, fracture of the tooth root may be experienced during extraction.

Differential Diagnosis (see pp. 48, 49)

This condition is considered to be different from osteogenesis imperfecta with dentinogenesis imperfecta, and consequently the name hereditary opalescent dentin is reserved for this condition. Radiographically it can be differentiated from dentinal dysplasia (4C36) by the absence of periapical radiolucencies and W-shaped roots.

Laboratory Aids

None.

Treatment

Restorative treatment is complicated by the fragility of the dentin. It may be necessary to reduce the tooth crown to the cervical margin and provide onlays and onlay dentures. The teeth are extremely friable to dental forceps.

Herpangina (3D42)

Herpangina is an acute, self-limiting infectious disorder caused by group A Coxsackie viruses, types 7, 9, and 16.

Clinical Features

The disorder is especially common during the summer in children up to age 6, although it may occur in persons up to 15 years of age or occasionally even older persons. After a 2- to 9-day incubation period (with 4 days being the average), the disease has a rapid onset with sore throat, dysphagia, hyperpyrexia, vomiting, headache, generalized muscle pain, and regional lymphadenitis. In the mouth, vesicles appear on the soft palate, uvula, and fauces. The oropharynx may be erythematous. Vesicles rupture, forming shallow, discrete ulcers 1 to 2 mm in diameter that persist for a period of 2 to 6 days. The disease usually resolves in from 2 to 6 days.

A few cases have been reported to be complicated by acute parotitis, meningitis, or hemolytic anemia.

Differential Diagnosis (see p. 38)

Only a small percentage of cases of herpangina are recognized, because the infection frequently takes a nonspecific or abortive course. Chicken pox, herpetic stomatitis, aphthous stomatitis, bacterial pharyngitis, and erythema multiforme should be considered in the differential diagnosis.

Laboratory Aids

The clinical signs and symptoms are usually sufficient for diagnosis. However, serologic tests for virus-neutralizing and complement-fixing antibodies may be performed. The virus can be isolated from hamsters or mice after inoculation of scrapings from the throat or oral lesions.

Treatment

No specific treatment is required. Bed rest and soft diet are recommended.

Herpes Simplex, Primary (1C31; 2E58; 3B17)

Primary herpes simplex is an acute vesicular, infectious disease, produced in humans by two strains of an ectodermotropic virus. Herpes hominis type 1 produces acute herpetic gingivostomatitis, and Herpes hominis type 2 produces herpes genitalis.

Clinical Features

The primary infection almost invariably occurs between 1 and 5 years of age. Adults are occasionally affected. Systemic involvement includes high fever, dehydration, irritability, malaise, headache, nausea, dysphagia, and regional lymphadenitis.

Orally, acute herpetic gingivostomatitis is characterized by swollen gingivae, increased salivation, pain, and halitosis. The interdental papillae are quite characteristic, presenting marked hypertrophy and erythema. Shortly thereafter, vesicles 2 to 4 mm in diameter develop on the gingival, lingual, labial, and buccal mucosa. The palate, pharynx, and tonsils may be affected as well. The vesicles are round to oval, sharply demarcated, and yellowish. The vesicles tend to coalesce, and within a few hours they rupture, forming shallow painful erosions covered by a yellow pseudomembrane with an erythematous margin.

Within 10 to 14 days the lesions heal spontaneously without scar formation. Recurrence of the primary form is extremely rare; when it occurs in older patients, leukemia or an immunodeficient condition should be suspected.

In herpetic conjunctivitis, edema and hyperemia of the palpebral conjunctiva, keratitis, ulceration of the cornea, and vesicles of the eyelids develop rapidly.

Inoculation herpes simplex is commonly seen in physicians, dentists, and dental hygienists. Initial manifestations generally involve the skin, the virus having entered a previous wound or abrasion.

Herpetic eczema is a herpetic infection superimposed on primary eczema. The condition is most often seen in young children and infants. Generalized skin involvement is the prominent feature.

Differential Diagnosis (see pp. 10, 25, 36)

Most vesicular diseases should be considered, as should burns, aphthous stomatitis, and food or drug allergies.

Laboratory Aids

In Paul's test, inoculation of salivary extract from affected patients onto the cornea of the rabbit will produce typical dendritic keratosis in 24 to 48 hours. Increased antibody titers will be observed in the patient's serum. Biopsy or smear from the base of an intraoral vesicle will demonstrate characteristic cells with ballooning degeneration. Another finding is the presence of intranuclear inclusions known as Lipschütz's bodies.

Treatment

The treatment is essentially palliative. Soft diet and rest are recommended. Mouth wash and maintenance of oral hygiene are essential in order to avoid superimposed infection. Corticosteroids should not be used, because they eliminate the inflammatory response essential to the production of antibodies (interferon) that will eventually control the viremia. Idoxuridine, which is a metabolic analogue of thymidine, is used with relative success to control recurrent ocular lesions. Its use in recurrent herpes simplex is also recommended, provided the treatment is started very early in the course of the disease.

Herpes Simplex, Recurrent (1C34)

Recurrent, or secondary, herpes simplex is a recurrent herpetic infection that may be precipitated by factors such as exposure to sunlight, fever, pregnancy, trauma, allergy, menstruation, mental or physical stress, gastrointestinal disturbances, and upper respiratory tract infections.

Clinical Features

The initial symptoms include a burning sensation, swelling, and soreness at the site where vesicular lesions will appear. Clear vesicles develop in small confluent groups, generally at the vermilion border of the lips. They are limited in number and soon rupture, becoming covered with a brownish yellow crust. Pustular formation is also frequent. Lesions of the eyes (keratitis) and genitalia also can occur. Intraoral lesions are extremely rare but may occur on the gingiva or hard palate. Regional lymphadenitis is absent. Recurrent lesions usually appear in the same area. A cyclic pattern has been observed. The lesions heal without scar formation in from 4 to 15 days.

Differential Diagnosis (see p. 10)

Impetigo, herpes zoster, and syphilitic chancre of the lip should be considered. Intraoral lesions should be differentiated from recurrent aphthous ulceration.

Laboratory Aids

Laboratory procedures are similar to those described for the primary form of the disease. Antibody titers in the primary disease are low initially and rise in about 10 days. In secondary infections the initial titer is high.

Treatment

Treatment is the same as for primary herpes simplex.

Histiocytosis X (3A6; 3A12; 5B23; 5C36)

The name histiocytosis X groups the entities clinically known as Letterer-Siwe's disease, Hand-Schüller-Christian's disease, and eosinophilic granuloma of bone. The conditions are grouped under the same name because all three are characterized histologically by marked proliferations of histiocytes. These conditions are of unknown etiology and can affect not only bone but also soft tissues, lymph nodes, and various organs, especially those associated with marked reticuloendothelial activity.

Clinical Features

Letterer-Siwe's disease (3A6) can be considered the acute manifestation of histiocytosis X. It invariably affects infants. Clinical findings include skin rash scattered over the trunk and the scalp and less severely over the extremities. High temperature, malaise, and irritability are also observed. Liver and spleen enlargement, as well as lymphadenopathy may be found early in the course of the disease. A number of organs and systems can be affected (e.g., spleen, liver, and lymph nodes). Bones are generally affected in the later periods of the disease. Anemia and other blood disorders can be present as a consequence of alteration in the reticuloendothelial system. Intraoral manifestations are characterized by the formation of intrabony granulomas that produce loosening of erupted teeth or premature exfoliation of tooth buds in infants up to age 6 months. Alveolar bone resorption is also evident, and granulomas can also develop in soft tissues, especially in the buccal mucosa. In very young children the disease progresses rapidly and is generally fatal. However, if there is some response to therapy the patient can be maintained for a number of years, eventually becoming an example of Hand-Schüller-Christian's disease.

Hand-Schüller-Christian's disease (3A12; 5C36) is considered the chronic form of histiocytosis X, generally affecting infants and young children. However, adolescents and adults are also affected. In this variety bone manifestations are much more marked, characterized by punched-out areas of destruction especially in the cranial bones, giving rise to the so-called geographic cranium. Several bones may be involved at the same time, including long bones, ribs, and others. The skin, liver, and spleen as well as lymph nodes are less frequently affected than in Letterer-Siwe's disease. Granulomas in the retroorbital region produce exophthalmus. Diabetes insipidus may ensue because of lesions in the hypophysis. Otitis media also may be present due to granulomas in the mastoid area. The oral lesions are the initial manifestations in about 30% of cases. The gingiva is often ulcerated, necrotic, and hemorrhagic. The teeth become mobile and eventually exfoliate because of alveolar bone destruction. Radiographic appearance demonstrates a typical floating-tooth picture (as in 5E36). The prognosis is poor, but patients generally follow a chronic course over a period of many years.

Eosinophilic granuloma (5B23) is considered a benign, localized manifestation of histiocytosis X. Generally, it affects young adults, and the lesions are present only in bone. Nearly any bone of the skeleton can be involved, but the majority of the lesions occur in the craniofacial bones. Two bones can be affected at the same time. Oral manifestations are generally confined to the molar area and the angle of the mandible. Tooth mobility and exfoliation of teeth are the chief complaints. If the cause of tooth loss is not properly diagnosed, the granulomatous tissue will extend to the neighboring areas, resulting in marked bone destruction and tooth exfoliation.

Differential Diagnosis (see pp. 35, 36, 60, 61)

Letterer-Siwe's disease should be differentiated from acute leukemia and other types of blood dyscrasias. Differentiation is easily achieved by means of complete blood and bone marrow examination. Ewing's sarcoma should also be differentiated from this generalized form of the disease. Hand-Schüller-Christian's disease, when it occurs in adults, should be differentiated from multiple myeloma. Either of these two conditions occurring in childhood should be differentiated from a large number of entities associated with premature loss of teeth and gingival hemorrhage. Proper clinical history and some laboratory analysis will contribute to the proper diagnosis. In young adults eosinophilic granuloma needs to be differentiated from cysts, osteomyelitis, various malignant lesions, and chronic inflammatory process.

Laboratory Aids

Biopsy of one of the granulomatous lesions will demonstrate a profusion of histiocytes accompanied by a variable amount of polymorphonuclear eosinophils, which are the salient histologic features in these three conditions. The final diagnosis of each of the varieties needs to be made by correlating the clinical findings with the histologic picture.

Treatment

Treatment for Hand-Schüller-Christian's disease and Letterer-Siwe's disease is in the hands of the physician. Several procedures are employed, including radiation therapy and some chemicals. Eosinophilic granuloma of bone is very susceptible to low doses of radiation therapy.

Hypercementosis (5C29)

Hypercementosis is an idiopathic overgrowth of cementum.

Clinical Features

The condition is usually discovered on routine roentgenographic examination as an asymptomatic radiopacity involving the apical one-third of a tooth. Hypercementosis is a smooth, ellipsoid swelling demarcated by a fine periodontal membrane space and lamina dura. The knoblike excrescence can prove a complication to dental extraction.

Differential Diagnosis (see p. 60)

True cementoblastoma has a more spherical appearance, and its calcific masses have a radiated appearance. Periapical cemental dysplasia also should be differentiated.

Laboratory Aids

None.

Treatment

None.

Hyperkeratosis (2B20; 2B21; 2D39) and Leukoplakia (1D39; 3E50)

The name hyperkeratosis implies an overproduction of keratin such that it is observed in areas where keratin normally does not occur (e.g., over most of the oral mucosa). Here, the name leukoplakia is used to connote a clinical white patch that cannot be rubbed off. No histologic definition is ascribed to it.

Clinical Features

These white lesions of the oral mucosa can be observed in any area, such as the buccal mucosa, lateral border of the tongue, floor of the mouth, palate, and lip. Clinically, they are characterized by irregular areas of whitening that cannot be rubbed off. Sometimes these areas of whitening are speckled with intercrossing areas of normal-looking mucosa. The etiology of this lesion is generally traumatic. Several forms of trauma could cause the formation of this whitening. The lesions are generally asymptomatic and may be discovered on routine examination, or the patient may accidentally see them and be curious about their nature. Tobacco in various usages can also produce hyperkeratosis (p. 169). Snuff hyperkeratosis manifests as an irregular silvery-white area, present only in those mucosal surfaces in contact with tobacco. Malignant transformation can occur as in 2B22.

Differential Diagnosis (see pp. 23, 24; 11, 38)

The differential diagnosis of white patches of the oral cavity includes all lesions that present in that form, including simple reactive hyperkeratosis, premalignant lesions, lichen planus, infection with *Candida albicans*, and some genodermatoses such as white sponge nevus and intraepithelial benign dyskeratosis.

Laboratory Aids

It is important that these lesions be biopsied. Under the microscope the final classification will be achieved; that is, plain lesions characterized by hyperproduction of orthokeratin or parakeratin with no other changes within the epithelial tissue will be distinguished from lesions with frank premalignant or malignant transformation. Therefore, biopsy of these lesions, especially in individuals over 40 years of age, should be a routine procedure.

Treatment

Surgical excision of the area of whitening is the indicated treatment.

Hyperplastic Frenulum (3A1)

The various oral frenulae are normally attached below the mucogingival junction. Hyperplastic frenulum, involving higher attachment of frenulae through the marginal or attached gingiva, may result in a fibrous band separating teeth and causing diastema (as in 3A1) or, by exerting tension on the gingiva, may contribute to the formation of periodontal pockets and Stillman's clefts. The lesion is a developmental abnormality.

Clinical Features

An asymptomatic hypertrophic band of fibrous connective tissue can be found gaining attachment most commonly on the labial aspect of the midline between the upper central incisors. The tissues may be blanched by pulling on the band. Complications arising from this condition are the formation of a diastema and abnormal space between the upper central incisors by tension and deprivation of the vasculature. Frenulae in relation to a periodontal lesion may exacerbate this condition.

Differential Diagnosis (see p. 35)

None.

Laboratory Aids

None.

Treatment

Surgical repositioning of the frenum is indicated.

Hypohidrotic Ectodermal Dysplasia (4A5 and 4A6)

The major components of hypohidrotic (anhidrotic) ectodermal dysplasia are hypodontia, hypotrichosis, and hypohidrosis. Principally affected are structures of ectodermal origin. The syndrome is usually transmitted as an X-linked recessive condition. Therefore, the majority of affected persons are males. However, a great number of females have manifested the complete syndrome. The increased parental consanguinity in these cases suggests autosomal recessive inheritance and illustrates the genetic heterogeneity of this syndrome.

Clinical Features

The face is quite characteristic, and affected individuals look enough alike to be mistaken for siblings. The skull resembles an inverted triangle. Marked frontal bossing, depressed nasal bridge (simulating the saddle nose of congenital syphilis), protuberant lips, and obliquely inserted ears are the most prominent features. Linear wrinkles are seen about the eyes and mouth.

The most striking oral finding is oligodontia, or in some cases, anodontia. The few teeth that may be present, generally incisors and canines, have a conical crown form. The alveolar process will not develop in the absence of teeth, resulting in loss of vertical dimension with consequent protruding lips.

Hypohidrotic ectodermal dysplasia may not be clinically manifested until the second year of life, and, because the physical features are not readily apparent, the child may appear to have a fever of unknown origin. The inability to sweat, due to marked aplasia of the eccrine sweat glands, results in intolerance to heat, with severe hyperpyrexia. The skin is soft and thin, presenting severe dryness, due to diminished numbers of sebaceous glands. Small hyperkeratotic plaques are frequently noted on the palms and soles.

At birth, the body is devoid of lanugo hair; after puberty, the beard is generally normal, but axillary and pubic hair is scant. The scalp hair is generally blond, fine, stiff, and short. The eyelashes and especially the eyebrows are often entirely missing. The fingernails and toenails are usually normal or slightly spoon shaped.

Differential Diagnosis (see p. 47)

Dominant hidrotic forms of ectodermal dysplasia are different syndromes from the one considered here. Progeria and congenital syphilis should be included in the differential diagnosis.

Laboratory Aids

The ability to sweat is easily demonstrated by employing the starch-iodine test. Other methods are available, such as agar plates with silver nitrate and potassium chromate, and $\emptyset$-phthalaldialdehyde in xylene. Sweat pore counts using dental rubber base can also be performed.

Treatment

Extraction of the few abnormal teeth is recommended, together with construction of full-mouth dentures. Dentures should be changed according to the growth of the patient.

Infectious Mononucleosis (3D41)

Infectious mononucleosis, a febrile condition affecting the lymphoreticuloen-dothelial system and the blood, is probably caused by the Epstein-Barr and other viruses.

Clinical Features

The oral finding of red palatal petechiae at the junction of the hard and soft palates is a reliable sign that appears by the second or third week of the course of the disease. Sore throat, acute gingivitis, and stomatitis, gray or white membranes, jaundice, and ulceration of oral tissues may also be found. Cervical nodes are involved, bilaterally.

The initial complaint generally includes sore throat, malaise, and light fever. Jaundice can also be seen, but most likely as a complication, after the second or third week of onset of the disease. In 50% of the patients the febrile stage lasts from 7 to 14 days.

Differential Diagnosis (see p. 37)

Herpangina and hand-foot-and-mouth disease should be considered on the basis of fever and similar location. Petechiae occur intraorally as manifestations of some blood dyscrasias and also as part of hereditary hemorrhagic telangiectasia and Fabry's syndrome.

Laboratory Aids

Blood analysis will demonstrate relative lymphocytosis with atypical lympho-cytes. The Paul-Bunnell test will show elevated agglutination of sheep erythro-cytes. This heterophil antibody reaction is a requirement for diagnosis.

Treatment

There is no specific treatment. Bed rest and proper (normal) diet are the indications of choice.

Lentigo Maligna Melanoma (3C36)

Lentigo maligna, or Hutchinson's malignant lentigo, is a superficially spreading, precancerous form of melanoma that by invasion becomes lentigo maligna melanoma.

Clinical Features

Intraorally, the early lesion, which may persist for several years, is an irregular, flat, spreading area of pigmentation varying in hue from tan to brown or black. Later, black nodules or a nodular pigmented (or nonpigmented) mass may grow rapidly, indicating melanoma. Occasional areas may be opalescent blue-gray and white, possibly representing regression of the lesion. The palate and gingiva are most commonly affected.

Relatively few intraoral examples have been reported, but these have had poor prognosis. On excision, recurrence should be anticipated in peripheral sites. Widespread lymph node and visceral metastases are usually terminal.

Differential Diagnosis (see p. 37)

The differential diagnosis is confined to lesions producing intraoral pigmentation.

Laboratory Aids

Biopsy is mandatory to establish an early diagnosis.

Treatment

The treatment of melanoma is controversial. However, the treatment of lentigo maligna of the skin by excision has a good prognosis. Consequently, an earlier diagnosis of intraoral lentigo maligna may reduce mortality from this condition. For melanoma, local excision, radical lymph node dissection, and various modalities of chemotherapy are currently being evaluated.

Leukemia, Acute Monocytic (2A9; 3B13)

Leukemia is a disease characterized by the appearance of immature neoplastic white blood cells in the circulation. A viral cause is considered probable but is as yet not fully proven.

Clinical Features

The different types of leukemia can produce oral manifestations, acute monocytic being the most frequent. The following clinical manifestations refer to acute monocytic leukemia.

Oral lesions in leukemia are characterized by hyperplastic gingivitis with a cyanotic bluish red discoloration. The lesions vary in degree and severity. In some patients there is diffuse enlargement of the gingiva. The oral tissues are friable and bleed easily. Frequently, hyperplastic gingivae may completely cover the teeth.

In severe cases, purpuric lesions and necrotic ulcerations of the oral mucous membranes are also seen. A nomalike complication may be associated with terminal cases of leukemia owing to lack of tissue defense against a minor irritant. Alveolar bone destruction and necrosis of the periodontal ligament may occasionally lead to loosening and exfoliation of teeth. Acute necrotizing ulcerative gingivitis may also be present.

The oral manifestations of leukemia result from both the basic systemic defect and local irritants. When the oral cavity is kept free of local irritants such as plaque, food debris, ill-fitting dentures, and the like, oral involvement may be minimal.

The course and complications of the disease depend upon the basic systemic defect. The condition generally has a fatal outcome.

Differential Diagnosis (see pp. 22, 36)

Other blood dyscrasias, as well as advanced periodontitis, necrotizing ulcerative gingivostomatitis, hyperplastic gingivitis, and noma, should be considered in the differential diagnosis.

Laboratory Aids

Hemogram and bone marrow examination establish the diagnosis. Gingival biopsy is only suggestive of the condition and must be corroborated by hematologic and/or bone marrow examination.

Treatment

The treatment is systemic and mostly palliative, encompassing a variety of means, such as chemotherapy, radiation therapy, bone marrow transplant, and some others. Several patients with acute myelogenous leukemia have achieved more than 3 years' survival after treatment with full-body radiation followed by transplant of genetically compatible bone marrow.

Lichen Planus (2B19; 2E53; 2E54)

Lichen planus is the most frequent dermatologic disease presenting oral involvement. The cause is unknown.

Clinical Features

The condition has a moderate predilection for females. In 30% to 40% of patients, oral manifestations are associated with skin lesions. In 25% of patients, only oral lesions are present.

A variety of patterns may occur in lichen planus, including reticular, annular, and plaquelike lesions and occasionally erosive, atrophic, bullous, or verrucous lesions.

Oral lesions occur most frequently on the buccal mucosa, the tongue, the gingiva, and the lips. A reticular pattern, formed by interlacing hyperkeratinized strands known as Wickham's striae, can be observed in most cases. The condition is usually symptomless, although some patients may complain of a burning sensation or metallic taste, especially in cases of bullous lichen planus. Skin lesions are bluish silver and are generally accompanied by pruritus. The genital mucosa also may be affected.

The disease may last for several days, weeks, or months. Recurrences are common. The erosive variety tends to remain for life and at times may become secondarily infected. Squamous cell carcinoma has been occasionally reported in a preexisting lichen planus, especially one of the erosive type.

Differential Diagnosis (see pp. 23, 25)

Leukoplakia, moniliasis, pemphigus, syphilis, erythema multiforme, chronic discoid lupus erythematosus, and recurrent aphthous ulceration should be included in the differential diagnosis. The bullous and erosive types should be differentiated from all the vesiculobullous disorders, including pemphigus vulgaris.

Laboratory Aids

Biopsy of an intraoral lesion generally will establish the final diagnosis. Direct and indirect immunofluorescent studies are indicated in the erosive variety in order to rule out other vesiculobullous disorders.

Treatment

The intraoral lesions as a rule are not treated. In severe cases, especially in the erosive variety, treatment with corticosteroids is indicated.

Linea Alba (2B16)

Linea alba is considered a variation within the normal range and, therefore, does not represent a true pathologic entity.

Clinical Features

Linea alba is a bilateral white line located on the buccal mucosa that follows the plane of occlusion of the teeth.

Differential Diagnosis (see p. 22)

Care should be taken not to confuse linea alba with other white lesions of the oral cavity.

Laboratory Aids

None.

Treatment

The condition is innocuous and requires no treatment.

Lingual Varicosities (2D46)

Varicosities can be observed in other oral locations but they are most frequently found on the ventral surface of the tongue, as lingual varicosities.

Clinical Features

This change in veins is observed in individuals generally 50 years of age and older; it represents an aging process. These varicosities most likely affect the ranine veins as well as some other minor veins in the area. Clinically, they are characterized by a rasimose proliferation of a deep purple color. If they occur in younger individuals, they might be interpreted as a premature aging phenomenon. There are no known systemic abnormalities or pathologic processes associated with this change.

Differential Diagnosis (see p. 24)

Telangiectasia in Rendu-Osler-Weber's syndrome could be confused with this condition in this particular location. The absence of other lesions will establish the differential diagnosis.

Laboratory Aids

None.

Treatment

None.

Lip Licking (1C25)

Lip licking is a consequence of maceration of the perioral skin due to chronic moistening of the lips by the tongue. This may be habit or factitial injury and may be exacerbated by secondary *Candida albicans* infection.

Clinical Features

The typical clinical finding is a circumoral erythema with fine cracks or desquamations found in affected children. The lesion will heal spontaneously, provided the habit is interrupted.

Differential Diagnosis (see p. 10)

The lesion is differentiated from erysipelas by its lack of brawny edema, induration, and fever.

Laboratory Aids

None.

Treatment

Zinc oxide or antifungal ointments may be applied until the habit is broken.

Lupus Erythematosus (1D38)

Lupus erythematosus is a multisystem disease of autoimmune origin that may affect many organs, in which case it is called systemic lupus erythematosus (SLE). It may, however, involve only a few tissues in the form of chronic discoid lupus erythematosus (DLE).

Clinical Features

Females are more frequently affected, with a female-to-male ratio of 10 to 1. The majority of patients are between 30 and 45 years of age. SLE and DLE present oral manifestations that are quite similar. Therefore, only the oral lesions of DLE will be described.

Round, well-circumscribed lesions can be seen on the vermilion border of both lips, with elevated margins and occasional areas of ulceration. The oral lesions of DLE are, as a rule, painless. Intraorally they occur in the buccal mucosa, the palate, and the tongue, in that order of sequence. They appear as rounded, slightly elevated plaques formed by white-blue, radial striae on an erythematous base. The radial appearance is quite characterstic for oral lesions of DLE. Rarely, ulceration may supervene.

Systemic manifestations of SLE can include, over any period of the patient's observation, butterfly erythematous eruption of the face, Raynaud's phenomenon, photosensitivity, alopecia, arthritis, pleuritis, and pericarditis, as well as other less frequent manifestations.

Differential Diagnosis (see p. 11)

Intraoral lesions of SLE and DLE should be differentiated from a variety of white lesions. Lichen planus especially, because of its similar white striated appearance, should be ruled out by biopsy.

Laboratory Aids

Biopsy of an intraoral lesion of lupus erythematosus will show atrophy of the overlying epithelium, a marked inflammatory infiltrate in the connective tissue, and also a characteristic perivascular inflammatory infiltrate mostly composed of lymphocytes and occasional plasma cells.

The periodic acid Schiff (PAS) staining reaction shows a thick, homogeneous, eosinophilic, PAS-positive band at the level of the epithelial basement membrane, which is considered quite typical and of diagnostic value for lesions of DLE. This change indicates an apparent thickening of the basement membrane caused by accumulation of fibrin and immunoglobulins. Deposits of immunoglobulins and complement have been demonstrated at the basement membrane zone in all oral lesions in both DLE and SLE as areas of granular fluorescence.

The LE test is the oldest and most highly specific test (effective in 85% of cases) to detect antibodies to nuclear components. Normocytic anemia will be detected in peripheral blood examination in the majority of patients with SLE. In the evaluation of patients with suspected lupus erythematosus, it is advisable to use the full array of specific laboratory procedures.

Treatment

The treatment is systemic, basically by means of corticosteroids or immuno-suppressive agents. Patients with either SLE or DLE should be referred to an internist for total evaluation and treatment.

Lymphadenitis (1E59, 1E60)

Nonspecific lymphadenitis of the cervicofacial nodes is an inflammation secondary to a source of infection or inflammation anywhere in the facial skin or scalp, the upper respiratory tract, the mouth, or the pharynx. Abscess, ulceration, acute necrotizing ulcerative gingivitis, acne vulgaris, traumatic ulcers, and dental infections are the most common causes. Lymphadenitis may also be secondary to infection within the bones of the skull, the salivary glands, the fascial planes, or the external ear.

Clinical Features

Occasionally single but sometimes multiple nodes in the submental, submandibular, or superficial cervical chain are most commonly affected. The nodes are slightly increased in size and are palpable, tender, and movable. Lymphadenitis may be accompanied by general symptoms such as lassitude, malaise, and fever. The onset of lymphadenitis has a temporal relation to the appearance of the source of the infection and generally runs a course of 7 to 10 days from the onset of the primary lesion. After the initial cause has been resolved, the lymphadenitis regresses spontaneously. Rarely, formation of an abscess within the lymph node may occur. In about 20% of the population a facial node (as in 1E60) is present slightly above the lower border of the mandible just anterior to the insertion of the masseter muscle where the facial artery, vein, and lymphatics cross the lower border of the mandible. Inflammation of this node gives rise to a tender swelling that has an apparent relation to the periapical areas of the lower molar and premolar teeth. Occasionally, this node may even be higher in the cheek. It is important to differentiate this from a dental infection.

Differential Diagnosis (see p. 12)

The differential diagnosis can include a great variety of lesions proper to either lymph nodes (i.e., infections, mononucleosis, cat-scratch disease, lymphatic neoplasia) or cysts and tumors of the neck. Metastasis can also be included, depending on the particular case.

Laboratory Aids

None.

Treatment

Treatment of the primary source of inflammation or infection will usually result in resolution of the lymphadenitis.

Lymphangioma (2A1; 2D47)

The lymphangioma is a benign neoplasm of lymphatic vessels.

Clinical Features

The lymphangioma is less common than the hemangioma and, as in hemangioma, the majority of cases are present at birth. These neoplasms do not have a sex predilection. When developing in the oral regions, they can be seen in the lips, the buccal mucosa, the tongue, and other areas, including the palate. The most common site is the tongue. Lesions can be single or multiple, most likely the latter. They can have the normal color of the oral mucosa (as in 2A1) or can be formed by rasimose proliferations having a port wine color (as in 2B47). The lesions are painless, and they do not change in size. Occasionally lymphangiomas in the tongue can grow to very large proportions, producing macroglossia. The same is true of lymphangiomas on the lips.

Differential Diagnosis (see pp. 21, 24)

The differential diagnosis should include hemangioma, multiple mucosal neuromas, Rendu-Osler-Weber's syndrome, and multiple neurofibromas.

Laboratory Aids

Biopsy of the lesion will confirm its vascular nature.

Treatment

The treatment of lymphangioma is surgical excision. These lesions are not amenable to radiation therapy. Recurrence can be as high as 50%.

Lymphoepithelial Cyst (2C28)

The so-called oral tonsils are lymphoid aggregates located in different areas of the oral cavity, especially on the dorsum of the tongue posterior to the vallate papilla and on the floor of the mouth. Cystic transformation of these lymphoid aggregates give rises to the so-called lymphoepithelial cyst. This cystic transformation can be explained on the basis of two possible mechanisms. Salivary gland epithelium may become entrapped within the lymphoid aggregates, or these lymphoid aggregates may present crypts lined by epithelium reaching deep into the lymphoid component. Secondary inflammation of these oral tonsils is often associated with obstruction of the crypt opening. When this occurs, the keratin normally produced by the epithelium accumulates, distending the cryptic space.

Clinical Features

In either event, a cystic transformation is characterized by a slow-growing, very well circumscribed, round mass that is yellowish in color. This mass is of variable size and is occasionally tender. The condition may be observed at any age.

Differential Diagnosis (see p. 23)

When the cyst is located in the anterior part of the mouth, one needs to consider a sialolith in the excretory duct of the submandibular glands. Also, neoplastic pathology of a minor salivary gland should be considered. When the cyst is located on the tongue, some entities such as neurofibroma and granular cell myoblastoma could be considered because of the similarity in color, but these two entities generally occur in a more anterior location.

Laboratory Aids

Biopsy will confirm the diagnosis.

Treatment

Treatment can be accomplished with conservative surgery.

Major Aphthous Ulceration (2A7; 2C35)

Major aphthous ulceration (also known as periadenitis mucosa necrotica recurrens and as Sutton's disease) consists of recurrent ulcerations of the oral mucosa of unknown cause that heal with scar formation. At present, it is considered to be a severe form of the recurrent aphthous ulcer.

Clinical Features

The condition is characterized by a single or multiple (but generally not exceeding 10 in number), large ulceration that occurs in any area of the oral mucosa. As a rule, the gingiva is not affected. Large ulcers also may be located on the soft palate and anterior tonsillar pillars. Occasionally, the laryngeal and genital mucosae may be involved.

Three clinical stages can be recognized. The first stage is characterized by the appearance of single or multiple reddish nodules that range from 1 to 4 cm in diameter. After a few days the nodules undergo ulceration, marking the beginning of the second stage. The ulcers are superficial with indurated borders. Later they become covered with an adherent, gray pseudomembrane. Pain is marked, especially after ingestion of citrus fruits. Healing with scarring represents the third stage of the disease (as in 2A7). Subsequent fibrous adhesion may lead to limitation of the oral opening or amputation of the tip of the tongue. The regional lymph nodes are tender and palpable.

The disease lasts from 1 week to 3 or 4 months. Characteristic lesions of the three stages may occur simultaneously. The condition is recurrent, beginning its cycle anew within a few weeks to several months. In some patients, recurrences follow one another without interruption.

Differential Diagnosis (see pp. 22, 24)

All ulcerative diseases should be ruled out, including squamous cell carcinoma.

Laboratory Aids

Recently immunoflourescent studies have revealed the presence of complement 3 (C 3) in the vicinity of blood vessels. However, this finding is not specific for the condition.

Treatment

Treatment is essentially symptomatic, with local topical anesthesia in order to relieve the pain. Several medications have been tried, including corticosteroids (both local and systemic), with no apparent success.

Malignant Lymphoma (3E52; 5E59)

The name malignant lymphoma covers a group of malignant tumors of the lymphoreticuloendothelial system. Because lymphoid cells in varying degrees of differentiation may be encountered and because the histological picture may change with time, definitive diagnosis is difficult. There are several different ways of classifying malignant lymphomas.

Clinical Features

Lesions are usually multifocal, firm lumps or radiolucencies in bone. The lymphoid tissues are predominantly affected, though varieties of lymphomas are found in the skin and bone. Various cell types will spill over into the blood in the leukemias. The lesions are progressively destructive; fever, weight loss, anemia, and disorders of immunity with secondary infections are common. In the oral cavity malignant lymphoma may manifest as ulcerative lesions of the palate, the buccal mucosa, and the gingiva. Painless enlargements of the cervical lymph nodes and loosening of teeth and destruction of bone by diffuse radiolucent lesions occur. The behavior of these tumors varies somewhat with the histologic pattern; they may have an insidious or a rapidly malignant progression.

Differential Diagnosis (see pp. 38, 62)

A great variety of malignant lesions could be considered.

Laboratory Aids

Application of immunochemical techniques will in most instances identify the responsible lymphoid cell.

Treatment

Chemotherapy and radiotherapy are the treatments of choice. Local surgical removal is used for single neoplasms.

Mandibulofacial Dysostosis (1A6)

Mandibulofacial dysostosis is a syndrome inherited as an autosomal dominant with incomplete penetrance and variable expressivity. More than 300 cases have been described to date.

Clinical Features

The facial appearance reveals downward-sloping palpebral fissures, hypoplastic malar bones, deformed or malplaced pinnae, and a receding chin. A coloboma in the outer third of the lower lid is characteristic. A deficiency of cilia medial to the coloboma is also noted in half of the reported cases. Deafness due to defects in ossicles and absence of the external auditory canal is present in one-third of cases. Ear tags and blind fistulas have been reported from the tragus of the ear to the angle of the mouth. The nose often exhibits obliteration of the nasal-frontal angle with the bridge of the nose raised. Lack of malar development creates the impression of an enlarged nose. Hypoplasia of alar cartilages results in narrowing of the nares.

The mandible is nearly always hypoplastic. Roentgenographic studies reveal a more obtuse mandibular angle than normal. Also, the ramus may be deficient, and the body of the mandible may be markedly concave on the undersurface. Flat or aplastic coronoid and condyloid processes may be evident. The palate is high or cleft in more than 30% of the cases. The teeth may be maloccluded, and open bite may be present.

Differential Diagnosis (see p. 9)

Differential diagnosis should include dominantly inherited maxillofacial dysostosis, oculoauriculovertebral syndrome, and Nager's acrofacial dysostosis.

Laboratory Aids

None.

Treatment

Corrective surgery can be used for the facial defects.

Median Rhomboid Glossitis (2E49)

Median rhomboid glossitis is a red, nodular, denuded area in the midline of the dorsum of the tongue of inflammatory or developmental origin. For a long time this condition was thought to be an abnormality caused by persistence of the tuberculum impar during embryonic tongue development. Recent reports implicate *Candida albicans* in the etiology.

Clinical Features

The condition presents as a slightly raised, rhomboid, red, nodular elevation in the midline of the dorsum of the tongue just anterior to the circumvallate papillae. Its size is constant, approximately 0.5 to 2.5 cm in its greatest dimension. The lesion is usually asymptomatic and is most frequently found in adult males. No nodes are palpable. The paucity of lesions reported in children as compared to adults lends support to an inflammatory cause. A chronic course can be expected. In a recent study, patients with diabetes mellitus were found to have a higher incidence of median rhomboid glossitis.

Differential Diagnosis (see p. 25)

Developmental angiomas, either hemangioma or lymphangioma or both, may arise in this site. Squamous cell carcinoma has been reported at this site in two instances. Benign lingual thyroid usually occurs more posteriorly in the area of the foramen cecum and, if necessary, can be confirmed by radioactive iodine scan.

Laboratory Aids

Smears for *Candida albicans* should be done. Biopsy, rarely done, shows pseudoepitheliomatous hyperplasia with superficial epithelial atrophy, as well as increased vascularity and chronic inflammatory infiltrate in the connective tissue.

Treatment

Antifungal therapy is of benefit in some patients.

Melanotic Neuroectodermal Tumor of Infancy (3A5)

Melanotic neuroectodermal tumor of infancy is an embryonal neoplasm of neural crest origin. It is generally present at birth and contains nests of neural cells and melanin-forming cells.

Clinical Features

This single expansile neoplasm is usually found in the anterior maxilla of newborns or infants. The lesion has a dark bluish hue owing to the presence of melanin. Radiographically, it presents as an ill-defined radiolucency in the anterior maxilla which produces displacement of tooth buds. In most reported cases, the behavior is benign, though the lesion may be prone to recurrence. The case illustrated in 3A5 proved to have a more aggressive course with involvement of the base of the skull. This neoplasm has been reported occasionally in other areas, such as the mediastinum and the scapular region. The lesion is not encapsulated. Due to the infiltrative nature of its component embryonal cells, it is locally invasive, but it does not metastasize.

Differential Diagnosis (see p. 35)

The age of the patient and the color and location of the lesion are quite characteristic. Nevertheless, congenital epulis of the newborn, neuroblastoma, and some odontogenic tumors should be considered in the differential diagnosis.

Laboratory Aids

High urine levels of 3-methoxy-4-mandelic acid, or vanillylmandelic acid (VMA), have been recorded in patients with this tumor. VMA levels fall after surgical removal. Biopsy of the lesion is quite characteristic.

Treatment

Complete surgical removal is indicated.

Melanotic Pigmentation (2B14; 4C30; 4D47 and 4D48)

Physiologic melanin deposition is found in the oral cavity in varying degrees according to racial extraction. Idiopathic pigmentation (melanosis) has a different distribution and may occur in sites liable to trauma. The hormonal changes of pregnancy and oral contraception may also give rise to pigmentation, as may abnormalities in corticosteroid metabolism in Addison's disease. Certain drugs, such as quinine derivatives, also can give rise to hyperpigmentation.

Clinical Features

Physiologic pigmentation is usually most marked on the attached gingiva as a symmetrical brown, blue, or black band that follows the wavy contour of the gingiva (as in 4C30; 4D47 and 4D48).

Differential Diagnosis (see pp. 22, 48, 49)

The differential diagnosis should be established with respect to several causes of intraoral pigmentation. Special consideration should be given to lead poisoning, which manifests with a dark bluish gingival band, and Addison's disease. Malignant melanoma does not present such a linear distribution, but it always should be considered in the differential diagnosis of intraoral pigmentation. Irregular macular patches of asymmetric distribution with no apparent cause (as in

2B14) may occasionally be found in Caucasians and would be clinically indistinguishable from hormonal or drug-induced hyperpigmentation, though the latter may also affect the palate. The correlation between the racial extraction of the patient and the lack of change in the gingival pigmentation is the best diagnostic indicator.

Laboratory Aids

None, but if Addison's disease is suspected, urinary steroids should be estimated over 24 hours.

Treatment

None.

Mesiodens (4A3)

Mesiodens probably arises from a supernumerary tooth bud derived from the germ of the permanent central incisor. Some authors have suggested clefting of a tooth bud. Mesiodens have been observed in siblings as well as in parents and offspring in several families. This could suggest an autosomal dominant mode of transmission with lack of penetrance in some families.

Clinical Features

Mesiodens is the most frequent supernumerary tooth and, as the term implies, is located in the maxillary midline between the two central incisors. The crown is almost always conical, though it may sometimes be inverted in position. It could be erupted or retained. Occasionally, when in the inverted position, it may erupt into the anterior portion of the floor of the nose. More than one mesiodens in the same patient has also been described.

The incidence of mesiodens among the Caucasian population has been stated to range from 0.1 to 1.0. It appears to be most frequent in males with a male-to-female ratio of 2 to 1.

Differential Diagnosis (see p. 47)

When the mesiodens is impacted, the differential diagnosis of odontoma should be considered. Once it has erupted, the diagnosis is self-evident.

Laboratory Aids

None.

Treatment

Surgical extraction is the usual treatment.

Metastatic Neoplasms (5C33; 5D37)

Metastic neoplasms are tumors arising from the spread of malignant neoplasms, most commonly from the breast, the lung, the kidneys, or the prostate and less frequently from other sites of origin.

Clinical Features

The presentation of metastasis in the jaw bones is variable, but it is most commonly observed as an osteolytic, single or multiple, ill-defined radiolucency. Some metastases provoke osteoblastic activity and are radiopaque. Prostate, breasts, and lung are the usual sites of origin of the radiopaque lesions. The molar-premolar mandibular area is the most commonly affected site. There may be swelling or expansion of the bone; teeth may be mobile and could be extracted in error. The patient experiences discomfort and dull pain. If the inferior dental nerve is invaded by the process, paresthesia or anesthesia of the lower lip will ensue. An occasional pathological fracture may also occur. Metastases indicate a late stage in the progress of the primary neoplasm, and consequently the patients have a poor prognosis.

Differential Diagnosis (see pp. 60, 61)

Malignant neoplasms primary to the area should be ruled out.

Laboratory Aids

With widespread bone metastases, serum calcium, phosphorous, and alkaline phosphatase may be elevated.

Treatment

Chemotherapy, radiotherapy, and sex hormone therapy in the case of breast and prostate tumors are indicated.

Minor Aphthous Ulceration (2A6)

Minor (recurrent) aphthous ulceration is a condition of the oral mucosa that is probably an abnormal immunologic hypersensitive reaction to an L-form streptococcus. This reaction is precipitated by such agents as trauma, psychologic stress, viruses, bacteria, autoimmune reaction, endocrine dysfunction, and allergy.

Clinical Features

The ulceration may be single or multiple and is usually recurrent. The lesions are extremely painful and generally preceded by a burning sensation. Any area of the oral mucosa may be affected, although the gingiva is generally spared. Occasionally, nonoral mucous membranes may be involved. The initial lesion is an erythematous area that soon becomes an ulcer 2 to 10 mm in diameter with an area of central necrosis. Later a thin, grayish pseudomembrane forms. The lymph nodes are tender and palpable. The ulcers heal without scarring within 1 or 2 weeks. In severe cases, eating may be impaired. Low-grade fever and malaise also may be present, especially if the aphthae are multiple.

Differential Diagnosis (see p. 21)

In primary herpetic stomatitis the gingivae are affected, and smears will show multinucleate giant cells. Depending on the patient's age, other ulcerative conditions should be included such as benign mucous membrane pemphigoid. A herpetiform variant of aphthous ulceration has been described in which as many as a hundred minute and very painful ulcers without erythematous rims are found on the lateral border of the tongue. This variant is probably viral, since inclusion bodies have been found in epithelial smears.

Laboratory Aids

No specific test is known. Histology is nonspecific.

Treatment

Topical escharotics, such as sodium bicarbonate, can effect symptomatic relief. Topical corticosteroids can be tried in severe cases.

Mucocele (2A5)

A mucocele results from rupture of a salivary gland duct, allowing the secretion to escape into the connective tissue. In some instances, obstruction may lead to retention of salivary secretion within the duct system, producing an epithelial-lined cyst.

Clinical Features

A mucocele usually appears suddenly on the oral mucosa as a semisolid, generally fluctuant, spherical mass. The lesion varies in size from a few millimeters to several centimeters in diameter. Its smooth glistening surface is usually translucent white or pink, but it may be blue and domed in some cases. Mucoceles may occur in association with minor salivary glands anywhere along the oral mucosa but are most commonly found on the mucous membrane of the lower lip. They are usually superficial lesions but may also occur in deeper submucosal tissue. Multiple mucoceles are observed occasionally. The lesion may continue to expand in size, rupture, and disappear, or it may recur. Recurrences are common with inadequate treatment.

Differential Diagnosis (see p. 21)

Clinical diagnosis usually presents no problem, although a deeper mucocele may occasionally simulate hemangioma or some other neoplastic lesion.

Laboratory Aids

Biopsy will demonstrate pools of mucus within a fibrovascular connective tissue. Occasionally the cavity is lined by epithelium. Adjacent minor salivary glands may show sialoadenitis and partial acinar necrosis.

Treatment

Surgery is the treatment of choice. Recurrences may require partial elimination of the affected gland.

Multiple Mucosal Neuromas, Medullary Carcinoma of the Thyroid, and Pheochromocytoma Syndrome (2D48)

The syndrome characterized by multiple mucosal neuromas, medullary carcinoma of the thyroid, pheochromocytoma, and marfanoid body build with muscle wasting of the extremities (sometimes known as multiple endocrinomatosis type III) is inherited as an autosomal dominant.

Clinical Features

The large, thick, nodular lips and thick, often everted upper eyelids form a distinct facies.

The mucosal neuromas usually involve the lips and the anterior one-third of the dorsal surface of the tongue. Occasionally, the buccal mucosa may also be affected. The mucosal neuromas are microscopically plexiform neuromas that usually appear in the first decade of life. These lesions are manifested as multiple, slightly elevated, shiny nodules that are easily movable. In addition to the labial and lingual neuromas, the nasal and laryngeal mucosae may also be affected. The thyroid carcinoma usually does not manifest itself until the second decade. It is found in more than 75% of affected individuals. Approximately 50% of affected patients present metastatic lesions at the time of first diagnosis. Almost 20% of the patients die as a consequence of metastasis from the thyroid carcinoma. The production of ACTH-like peptides by these neoplasms has been diagnosed in about half of affected individuals. The pheochromocytoma manifests either in the second or third decades of life and is usually multiple and frequently bilateral. Almost all affected individuals exhibit a marfanoid or asthenic body build. Muscle wasting of the extremities may resemble a myopathic state.

Differential Diagnosis (see p. 25)

Neurofibromatosis, Sipple's syndrome (medullary carcinoma with pheochromocytoma), Marfan's syndrome, and various mytotonic states should be included in the differential diagnosis.

Laboratory Aids

Early endocrine evaluation in patients with the oral manifestations of the syndrome is imperative in view of the high malignant potential of medullary carcinoma of the thyroid. Determination of plasma immunoreactive calcitonin, which is a hormone secreted by the thyroid carcinoma, will demonstrate the presence of even minute thyroid lesions. The presence of pheochromocytoma can be determined by evaluation of urinary levels of epinephrine, vanillylmandelic acid, and metanephrines. Histamine skin tests are also of diagnostic value. Biopsy of an intraoral lesion will demonstrate the plexiform neuroma.

Treatment

If the condition is diagnosed early in life, patients can be periodically monitored for immunoreactive calcitonin. Thyroidectomy is recommended as a preventive measure. The oral lesions are generally not treated.

Multiple Myeloma (5B21; 5C34 and 5C35)

Multiple myeloma is a malignant neoplasm of bone marrow in which monoclonal plasma cells produce multifocal tumors and hypergammaglobulinemia.

Clinical Features

The condition may present as a unilocular radiolucency (as in 5B21) or as multiple sharply punched-out radiolucencies, the commonest sites being the body, ramus, and angle of the mandible. There is usually bone pain, and teeth may become mobile. A deep sessile swelling may be present. If the teeth are removed, the socket fails to heal and a polypoid mass may make its appearance in the tooth socket. Men are twice as commonly affected as women. The lymph nodes may also be affected. Anemia and secondary amyloidosis may be present. Lesions are mostly observed in bones with a great hematopoietic capacity. The skull and long bones are invariably affected.

Differential Diagnosis (see pp. 60, 61)

Hand-Schüller-Christian's disease in the adult has been reported and should be differentiated.

Laboratory Aids

Serum electrophoresis will delineate the hypergammaglobulinemia and Bence-Jones's protein can be assayed in the urine.

Treatment

Palliative X-ray therapy and chemotherapy are used.

Multiple Nevoid Basal Cell Carcinoma Syndrome (1A11)

Multiple nevoid basal cell carcinoma syndrome presents as its major components multiple nevoid basal cell carcinomas, cysts of the jaws, and vertebral and rib anomalies, chiefly bifid rib. The syndrome is inherited as an autosomal dominant condition with high penetrance and variable expressivity.

Clinical Features

The face is characterized by mild hypertelorism, frontal and biparietal bossing, mild mandibular prognathism, and a broad nasal root. Rarely, strabismus and cataracts are present.

The main oral component is numerous odontogenic keratocysts of the maxilla and mandible. They may be as large as several centimeters in diameter and have a marked tendency to recur after surgical removal. Occasional transformation into ameloblastoma has been reported. The multiple odontogenic keratocysts can appear as early as age 5 or 6 years, interfering with the normal development of the permanent dentition. There is good evidence that the cysts are derived from the overlying oral epithelium.

The nevoid basal cell carcinomas generally appear in childhood or at puberty, involving the nose, eyelids, cheeks, trunk, arms, and neck. They are flesh colored to pale brown. Milia, epithelial inclusion cysts, lipomas, and fibromas are often intermixed with the skin carcinomas. Small pits in the palms and soles are also a component of the syndrome.

Mild mental retardation is noted in about 15% of affected individuals. Medulloblastoma has been reported in several instances, and in some families a sibling of an affected individual has died in early childhood of medulloblastoma. Skeletal anomalies include bifurcation or splaying of one or more ribs, shortened fourth metacarpal, bridging of the sellaturcica, spina bifida occulta in the cervicothoracic area, and kyphoscoliosis.

Differential Diagnosis (see p. 9)

Multiple cylindromas of the scalp, pseudohyperparathyroidism, epidermal nevus syndrome, and isolated multiple odontogenic keratocysts should be considered in the differential diagnosis.

Laboratory Aids

Biopsy of skin lesions or of the jaw cysts, together with the radiologic findings in the jaws and the chest, are conclusive for the diagnosis.

Treatment

Careful surgical removal of the odontogenic keratocyst in order to prevent recurrences is the treatment of choice. Skin lesions are treated by the dermatologist with different means, namely, surgery, cryosurgery, and the like.

Nasopalatine Cyst (5E60)

The nasopalatine cyst is a developmental cyst that occurs in the line of fusion between the two premaxillary bones. Therefore, it will be observed between the two maxillary central incisors at the level of the anterior incisive canal.

Clinical Features

The condition has been reported at all ages. It is generally an accidental radiographic finding. Occasionally, if it occurs in a more superficial location (in which case it is known by the name incisive papilla cyst), it erodes bone very slightly. In this instance it will be detected clinically as a swelling of the incisive papilla. When it occurs entirely within bone, it is, as a rule, asymptomatic. Radiographically, it has a typical heart shape. This configuration is produced by the projection of the anterior nasal spine into the cystic cavity. Other images, such as a frankly round or pear-shaped radiolucency, are also observed. Both sexes are affected equally.

Differential Diagnosis (see p. 62)

Periapical pathology associated with the central incisors should be considered in the differential diagnosis.

Laboratory Aids

None.

Treatment

Surgical excision is the treatment of choice.

Necrotizing Ulcerative Gingivostomatitis (3B18)

Necrotizing ulcerative gingivostomatitis is an acute or subacute oral inflammation primarily involving the free gingival margin, the crest of the gingiva, and the interdental papillae. The condition may occasionally spread to other areas of the oral mucous membranes. The classic etiologic concept—that the disorder is caused only by a symbiotic relationship between *Bacillus fusiformis* and *Borrelia vincentii* (Vincent's organisms)—is no longer tenable. Vibrios, hemolytic streptococci, certain viruses, and poor oral hygiene in combination are probably implicated, producing enzymes and toxins that cause necrotizing ulcerative gingivostomatitis. Mental stress also may play some role in the development of the disorder, as may smoking.

Clinical Features

The condition has its peak incidence during winter in patients in their early twenties, with a marked predilection for males. Children are rarely if ever affected. The initial lesions—swollen, red papillae—generally occur in the mandibular molar area. However, other gingival areas may be affected. The edematous gingiva rapidly undergoes ulceration, producing characteristic, punched-out erosions of the dental papillae. The free gingiva becomes covered with a yellowish gray pseudomembrane with a red halo. Fetor ex ore (halitosis) and excessive salivation are marked, and patients frequently complain of a metallic taste. Pain, tenderness, and bleeding lead to inability to eat. Regional lymphadenitis is usually marked. Low-grade fever, headache, and malaise are common. The condition may involve the oropharynx and other areas of the oral mucosa if the patient's resistance is low or the condition is not treated. In such patients, tachycardia, leukocytosis, and gastrointestinal disturbances may occur.

The condition has a rapid onset. If treated, it generally subsides within 48 hours. Spontaneous remission and healing also may occur in 1 to 3 weeks.

Recurrence of the disease is observed with high frequency, generally owing to retention of microorganisms and debris in the punched-out areas of destruction. Occasionally, considerable tissue destruction occurs, producing marked recession of the interdental papillae and of the marginal gingiva. Bone sequestration may occur. Rarely, complications such as noma, septicemia, and even death may occur.

Differential Diagnosis (see p. 36)

Blood dyscrasias and scurvy should be considered. Primary herpetic gingivostomatitis must not be confused with this entity. Acatalasia should be considered if the patient is of Japanese ancestry.

Laboratory Aids

The diagnosis is made clinically. Smears contain Vincent's organisms in large numbers.

Treatment

Oral penicillin or metronidazole are effective combined with curettage and rinsing with hydrogen peroxide.

Neurofibromatosis of von Recklinghausen (1A10)

Neurofibromatosis of von Recklinghausen is a syndrome consisting of multiple skin tumors and cutaneous pigmentation. The condition is inherited as an autosomal dominant. Its occurrence is estimated at 1 in 3,000 live births.

Clinical Features

The facial appearance is quite striking when the tumors develop on the skin of the face, especially the eyelids. Café-au-lait spots are also part of the facies. Less severely affected patients will present only a few or no neurofibromas of the facial skin.

Oral involvement is seen in about 7% of patients presenting single or multiple tumors. Tumors may affect any area of the oral cavity, but usually occur on the lateral borders of the tongue. The intraoral tumors are similar to those found on the skin; that is, they are neurofibromas of the plexiform type. Occasionally neurilemomas are seen associated with the condition, especially on the tongue. The skin tumors consist of neurinomas, soft fibromas, or most often neurofibromas. They may be present at birth or appear early in life and increase in number and size at puberty. They vary from pea-size growths to huge, pendulous growths. Malignant transformation of one or more of the neurofibromas occurs in a small percentage of patients.

Multiple café-au-lait pigmentations of the skin usually appear within the first decade and are present in 90% of affected individuals. Their color varies from yellowish to chocolate brown. Pigmentation generally precedes the tumors. Pigmentations occur most often about the axilla (the freckled axilla sign) and the waist, presenting a smooth contour. Neurofibromas can develop in nearly any area of the body, including intraosseous locations. Pheochromocytoma is occasionally found in patients with neurofibromatosis.

Differential Diagnosis (see p. 9)

Multiple lipomatosis and tuberous sclerosis, as well as other phacomatoses, should be included in the differential diagnosis. The multiple mucosal neuroma syndrome should also be considered.

Laboratory Aids

Biopsy of one of the cutaneous or intraoral neurofibromas is of diagnostic value.

Treatment

Surgical excision of the neurofibroma for aesthetic reasons is often accomplished. Malignant transformations are treated as are other malignancies.

Nicotinic Stomatitis (3D49)

Nicotinic stomatitis, also known as smoker's palate, is characterized by marked hyperkeratosis of the hard palate and secondary inflammation of underlying structures. It is seen in a considerable number of heavy tobacco smokers, including pipe smokers, cigar smokers, and cigarette smokers.

Clinical Features

The great majority of cases are seen in males with a mean age of 50 years. Most frequently affected are pipe smokers, followed by cigarette smokers, and, far behind, cigar smokers. The initial manifestation of the condition is marked erythema of the palate. This is followed by numerous papular elevations around the opening of the excretory ducts of the palatal minor salivary glands. These elevations, of various sizes, soon become covered with a white to gray, generally uniform layer of either orthokeratin or parakeratin formation. The lesion progressively extends to the rest of the hard palate. Occasionally, whitening can also be seen in the soft palate. With time, cracks and fissures appear in the palate, which then presents the late clinical picture of the condition, namely, elevated, keratinized nodules of various sizes each with a central, small, red, rounded point, representing the ductal opening of a minor salivary gland. The nodules are separated by the small fissures. The entire palatal surface, then, presents a rough, irregular appearance.

The thickness and general clinical appearance of the lesion vary according to the amount of tobacco used and the duration of the lesion.

Some authors have considered that this condition might become malignant. A histologic survey, performed by the authors in 66 cases of nicotinic palatal leukokeratosis, showed that one case presented epithelial histologic changes compatible with the diagnosis of premalignant epithelial dysplasia.

Differential Diagnosis (see p. 38)

The condition presents such a typical clinical appearance that differential diagnosis is essentially unnecessary. Nevertheless, hyperkeratosis of other causes could be considered. Reverse smoking, a frequent practice in some areas of India, also induces palatal changes but with more pronounced clinical manifestations and early malignant transformation.

Laboratory Aids

Biopsy should be performed in order to eliminate the possibility of malignant transformation.

Treatment

It is assumed that remission occurs when patients abandon the smoking habit.

Odontodysplasia (4D38)

Odontodysplasia, also known as ghost teeth, is a regional lack of tooth development of unknown etiology affecting enamel and dentin. However, local vascular abnormalities have been implicated because of the occurrence of nevus flammeus in the affected quadrant. Also, a viral etiology has been thought possible, owing to some virus that may become lodged in the odontogenic epithelium and interfere with proper tooth formation.

Clinical Features

Both deciduous and permanent teeth in any quadrant of the dental arch can be misshapen and have small roots with large apical foramina. The enamel, dentin, and cementum are hypoplastic. The pulps are readily exposed by caries. Radiographs will show poorly formed teeth. There is no proper demarcation between the different dental tissues. The overall appearance is that of hypocalci-fied, malformed teeth; hence the name ghost teeth.

Differential Diagnosis (see p. 49)

The radiologic appearance is quite characteristic, making diagnosis easy.

Laboratory Aids

None.

Treatment

Extraction and replacement of the teeth with an appropriate prosthesis is indicated.

Odontogenic Keratocyst (4E56; 5B22; 5D40)

The odontogenic keratocyst is considered by several investigators to be the same as or similar to the primordial cyst. The cystic cavity is lined by odonto-genic epithelium, which eventually produces parakeratin.

Clinical Features

This cyst can be single or multiple and it can occur at almost any age, with a mean age of 30 to 40 years. When multiple, it is associated with the multiple nevoid basal cell carcinoma syndrome. The majority of odontogenic keratocysts occur in the mandible, with only 20% developing in the maxilla. The most frequent site is the mandibular third molar area. The cyst has no particular clinical characteristics. It can be accompanied by pain or secondary infection, as can any other lesion of bone. Radiographically it can be unilocular or multi-locular. Root resorption of adjacent teeth can also be observed. One point to remember is that odontogenic keratocysts have a marked tendency to recur.

Differential Diagnosis (see pp. 50, 60, 61)

The differential diagnosis should include ameloblastoma, dentigerous cyst, and aneurysmal bone cyst, among others. If multiple, the multiple nevoid basal cell carcinoma syndrome (see p. 165) should be ruled out.

Laboratory Aids

Biopsy will reveal a cavity lined by an odontogenic epithelium demonstrating a basal cell layer in which the cells are arranged in a picket fence formation. Marked hyperchromatism and polarization of nuclei are also observed. The epithelium will be two or three rows in thickness, and the surface will present parakeratin formation in about 80% of cases.

Treatment

Surgical excision is the treatment of choice. Care must be taken to excise this cyst totally because, as mentioned above, it has a marked tendency to recur. Occasional transformation of this cyst into squamous cell carcinoma has been reported.

Odontogenic Myxoma (5D38; 5E54)

Odontogenic myxoma is a neoplasm that arises almost exclusively in the jaw. It is thought to be of mesenchymal origin, most likely derived from the dental papilla or the periodontal ligament. Myxomas of other bones are essentially unknown.

Clinical Features

This neoplasm is an expansile growth that occurs most frequently in the mandible. It does not present a sex predilection and is generally observed in patients between 20 and 40 years of age. It may be associated with an impacted tooth or with a missing tooth. Radiographically, it is characterized by a generally multiple radiolucency, which expands bone and may produce destruction of the cortex. A honeycomb appearance can also be observed. Teeth may be displaced by the neoplasm, and root resorption may be observed.

Differential Diagnosis (see pp. 61, 62)

The differential diagnosis should include a large number of tumors of the jaw, among them, ameloblastoma. Other nonneoplastic lesions such as fibrous dysplasia should also be considered.

Laboratory Aids

Biopsy will demonstrate the nature of the lesion.

Treatment

Surgical excision is recommended. Myxomas have a marked tendency to recur.

Odontoma (5C25; 5D45; 5E56)

Odontoma is considered a benign neoplasm derived from several odontogenic tissues. Some authors have considered odontoma to be a hamartoma and not a real neoplasm.

Clinical Features

Two varieties of odontoma are recognized, compound and complex. They share the feature of occurring at any age and in almost any location in the maxilla or mandible. They do not have a sex predilection. Compound odontoma (as in 5D45) is characterized by the abnormal formation of small denticles. These small teeth are essentially identical to normal teeth with the exception of their abnormal size and shape. Cementum, dentin, and enamel as well as pulp are arranged in the proper manner. The number of denticles can vary from a few up to several dozen. Radiographically they have a very typical appearance demonstrating the presence of the small teeth. The complex odontoma (as in 5C25; 5E56) is that variety in which the dental tissues are arranged in a haphazard fashion. Abnormal dentin, enamel, and cementum formation is observed intermixed with areas of apparently normal tissues. The arrangement of these tissues does not, however, form denticles as in compound odontoma. The complex odontoma can reach considerable proportions, and sometimes it is associated with an impacted tooth.

Differential Diagnosis (see pp. 60, 61, 62)

The compound odontoma, on radiograph, is quite evident; therefore, there is no need to establish a differential diagnosis. The complex odontoma can occasionally be confused with cementoma, fibrous dysplasia, and, in rare instances, osteogenic sarcoma. Multiple odontomas are occasionally observed in patients with Gardner's syndrome (see p. 127).

Laboratory Aids

Biopsy of either lesion is commonly employed. Histologic examination of the tissue will demonstrate the neoplasm.

Treatment

Surgical excision is the indicated treatment.

Ossifying Fibroma (5B17)

Ossifying fibroma is a benign central neoplasm predominantly of the mandible.

Clinical Features

The tumor presents as a solitary, painless, slow-growing, expansile, radiolucent lesion in the body of the mandible or adjacent to tooth roots. The neoplasm becomes increasingly calcified and flecked. Radiopacities appear centrally in the radiograph. Adjacent teeth may be displaced, but the lesion is usually well defined. The behavior of the neoplasm is usually benign; however, locally aggressive fibroosseous lesions have occurred in juveniles in the maxilla.

Differential Diagnosis (see p. 59)

A great variety of bone neoplasms such as osteoblastoma and osteoid osteoma and other lesions, such as fibrous dysplasia and central giant cell granuloma, should be considered.

Laboratory Aids

Diagnostic criteria for the separation of this lesion from fibrous dysplasia of bone and also from the so-called cementoossifying fibroma are a matter of personal histologic interpretation by the pathologist.

Treatment

The lesion should be removed conservatively by curettage since recurrences are rare.

Osteogenesis Imperfecta (5E50 and 5E51)

Osteogenesis imperfecta is inherited as an autosomal dominant; however, only about one-third of affected patients present a familial history of the condition. The remaining two-thirds consists of sporadic cases and a few patients with familial pedigrees that possibly suggest autosomal recessive inheritance. Those having a family history are inclined to have the disease in a milder form and to manifest it later in life. The degree of expressivity is variable. Only about one in three patients presents the complete syndrome.

Clinical Features

The skull is large, especially in the anteroposterior direction. The forehead is broad and bossed, with a temporal bulge. The eyes often present with blue sclerae, which may be the only expression of the syndrome. All bones are very fragile, and patients experience a variable number of fractures, including intrauterine fractures. Mental development is within normal limits. Somatic growth is impeded in patients experiencing numerous fractures and in patients with severe congenital forms. Roentgenographic examination of the skull reveals remarkably thin calvaria and the presence of numerous Wormian bones in the occipital region. The long bones are generally bowed or shortened. Twenty-five percent of affected patients have laxity of ligaments with resultant and persistent dislocation of joints. Deafness is frequent, beginning in the third decade. Progressive hearing loss ensues. Dentinogenesis imperfecta is seen in the primary dentition of about 80% of patients. The permanent teeth show similar changes in about 35% of patients. The degree of bone involvement appears to have no correlation to the degree of tooth involvement. The crowns of affected teeth are usually vertically smaller than normal. Subsequent to eruption, the dentition may be opalescent or translucent. As the patient ages, the teeth darken, and the enamel, which is normal, is lost because of the pathology in the underlying dentin. Roentgenographically, the roots of the teeth are thin and shortened, and pulp chambers are diminished or absent.

Differential Diagnosis (see p. 62)

Differential diagnosis should include hereditary opalescent dentin, cleidocranial dysplasia, pyknodysostosis, osteoporosis, Ellis-van Creveld's syndrome, achondroplasia, and Ehlers-Danlos's syndrome.

Laboratory Aids

Increased presence of alpha-III-type collagen in fibroblast cultures has been described in a small percentage of cases. Histologic examination of the teeth reveals a reduced degree of scalloping of the dentinoenamel junction. The dentin appears laminated and contains tubules of abnormal size and shape. Biochemical studies indicate diminished calcification manifested by zones of interglobular dentin.

Treatment

Treatment is still in the experimental stages. Fluoride and magnesium are being used as systemic therapy. Genetic counseling is imperative.

Osteoid Osteoma (5D46)

Osteoid osteoma is a benign neoplasm of bone. Some authors consider this condition an overreaction to trauma or inflammation.

Clinical Features

The lesion is rare in the maxilla or mandible. When it occurs, it has a predilection for the mandible and generally is observed in the first decade of life. Clinically it is characterized by intense pain disproportionate to the size of the lesion, which generally is very small. Soft tissues of the involved area can be swollen and tender. Males are affected twice as frequently as females. Radiologically, this condition is quite characteristic, presenting a central radiopaque nidus surrounded by an area of radiolucency.

Differential Diagnosis (see p. 61)

The differential diagnosis should include benign osteoblastoma as well as osteomyelitis and bone sclerosis.

Laboratory Aids

Biopsy will demonstrate the nature of the lesion.

Treatment

Surgical excision is the treatment of choice. Before surgery is undertaken, the patient is placed on regular doses of aspirin, which controls the marked pain accompanying the lesion.

Osteomyelitis (5D47)

Osteomyelitis constitutes an acute or chronic inflammation of bone marrow. A variety of pyogenic organisms may be responsible. Acute osteomyelitis is characterized by pus in the bone marrow, necrosis and sequestration of bone, peripheral sclerosis of bone, and subperiosteal proliferation of bone. The pus penetrates the bone to drain through multiple sinuses. Chronic osteomyelitis may be a prolongation of an acute inflammatory process over many years, with death of bone and sequestration that is very difficult to eradicate. A variety of osteomyelitis, chronic sclerosing osteomyelitis, is characterized by a subacute inflammation of the bone marrow and sclerosis of the bone.

Clinical Features

A rare form of acute osteomyelitis occurs in infants and young children. It is of hematogenous origin and affects the alveolar process of the maxilla, frequently with multiple sinuses around the deciduous teeth that discharge through the periodontal membrane. In adults, the mandible is more frequently involved, and the disease presents orally as an acute painful swelling with fever and cervical lymphadenopathy. Pus may discharge from sinuses in the buccal sulcus. A nonvital, tender tooth with a periapical abscess may be the cause. Fractures of the jaw may be secondarily complicated with osteomyelitis. Anesthesia or paresthesia of the inferior dental nerve may be found. Radiographically, the lesion shows as a diffuse radiopacity with focal areas of bone sclerosis, indicating sequestration. Osteomyelitis may develop in patients in whom the bone pattern is abnormal for any reason, including osteopetrosis, cemental dysplasias, Paget's disease of bone, and radionecrosis. The chronic suppurative osteomyelitis is frequently very resistant to treatment, and large areas may be lost by sequestration.

Differential Diagnosis (see p. 61)

Radiographically a moth-eaten appearance is quite characteristic. Nevertheless, Paget's disease of bone and cemental and fibrous dysplasias could be considered. The cause of the process should be established in order to institute proper diagnosis. Osteomyelitis of such unusual causes as tuberculosis can affect the jaws, as can some more common conditions such as actinomycosis.

Laboratory Aids

Pus should be sent for smear and culture. The white blood count will frequently be elevated, as will the erythrosedimentation rate.

Treatment

High doses of antibiotics prescribed for a prolonged period of time are necessary. Excision of sequestra and affected teeth and curetting of the bone may encourage healing. Fractures must be rigidly fixed.

Osteosarcoma (5C32; 5D41)

Osteosarcoma, also known as osteogenic sarcoma, is a malignant neoplasm of bone. Histologically it presents different stages of malignant bone formation. The different histologic typings and varieties of this entity will not be undertaken here since they do not represent a modification of prognosis and/or treatment.

Clinical Features

Osteogenic sarcoma generally occurs in individuals under 30. Males are more frequently affected than females. The tumor occurs most often in long bones, especially in the vicinity of the knee joint. Pain accompanies the lesion, as does clinical deformity of the affected area. A history of trauma previous to development of the tumor can generally be elicited. When the sarcoma is present in the facial region, the mandible is more frequently affected than the maxilla. The symptomatology is parallel to that of the long bones; that is, pain and swelling occur over the affected area with consequent loosening of teeth, paresthesia, and toothache. Again, one can elicit a history of trauma, but there is no relationship between trauma and the development of this tumor. Most likely the trauma has attracted attention to the area. Osteogenic sarcoma develops with a high frequency in patients affected by Paget's disease of bone (see p. 178). It also occurs with high frequency in patients whose bones have been irradiated for other purposes and in patients with retinoblastoma. Radiographically it can present as a radiopaque or radiolucent destructive mass. Basically, the tumor is bone forming, so at one time or another during the radiologic examination, spicules of bone formation can be observed. One of the typical radiologic findings described in association with this neoplasm is the so-called sunray appearance produced by thin spicules of bone growing at the periphery of the tumor. Illustrated in 5C32 is another radiologic finding, marked enlargement of the periodontal ligament. This finding is shared by several other malignant lesions and should be considered an indication of malignancy rather than an indication of a particular tumor. The neoplasm has a very rapid course, and the prognosis in the oral regions is very poor.

Differential Diagnosis (see pp. 60, 61)

The differential diagnosis should include a great variety of lesions associated with bone formation. The specificity of this particular neoplasm for a young age group and its characteristic rapid growth together with the radiologic appearance are quite indicative.

Laboratory Aids

Biopsy will indicate the malignant nature of the lesion.

Treatment

The treatment of choice is radical surgery. Radiation therapy is contraindicated. The prognosis is very poor with the 5-year survival rate fluctuating between 15% and 20%.

Paget's Disease of Bone (5A2, 5A3, 5A4, and 5A5)

Paget's disease of bone, also known as osteitis deformans, is a disease of unknown etiology affecting multiple bones. Some authors have proposed a vascular etiology for this condition based upon increased vascularity with vessels similar to those in arteriovenous aneurysm. This etiology is also based upon the fact that, histologically, the stroma in bone lesions of patients with Paget's disease have a marked degree of vascularization.

Clinical Features

The condition is seen in individuals over 40 years of age, with a slight predilection for males. Almost all bones can be involved. The major characteristic is enlargement of the affected bone. In about 50% of cases, there is involvement of jaw bones, with marked predilection for the maxilla. The most frequent complaint is bone pain, severe headache, deafness due to compression of the cochlear nerve, blindness due to compression of the optic nerve, dizziness, and weakness. A frequent complication is development of either osteogenic sarcoma or true giant cell tumor of bone. Another complication of the bone lesions is spontaneous fracture. In the jaw, fracture as well as osteomyelitis can be associated with dental pain. Bowing of legs is very marked and of diagnostic aid. When in the jaw, the lesion can be observed initially in either the maxilla or mandible, most likely the maxilla. In many cases, the condition is confined to the maxilla for a period of time before it manifests in some other bones. Maxillary and mandibular manifestations are characterized by generalized enlargement of these bones with consequent tooth diastema due to migration of teeth. If the patient is edentulous, a generalized enlargement of either the maxillary or mandibular alveolar ridges can be observed. In this case, the main complaint of the patient will be the inability to wear the old dentures. The disease has a slow, chronic course. Radiographically, it is characterized by the presence of areas of radiopacity alternating with areas of radiolucency, an appearance described as cotton wool. In the area of the maxilla and mandible this cotton wool manifestation is accompanied by areas of hypercementosis. This radiologic appearance can be confused, in those cases confined to the jaw, with periapical cemental dysplasia. The radiologic appearance portrays the basic pathologic process, resorption and softening of bone, represented by the radiolucent areas, and dysplastic new bone formation not related to functional requirements, represented by areas of marked radiopacity. Both stages can occur either simultaneously or alternatively. The cotton wool appearance can be observed in other bones, especially those of the skull.

Differential Diagnosis (see p. 59)

If the attending physician or dentist has a detailed clinical history as well as several radiographs and laboratory values as explained below, the diagnosis is quite evident. Nevertheless, in those cases that originate in the maxilla or mandible, periapical cemental dysplasia, familial autosomal cemental dysplasia, sclerosing osteitis, cementoma, and florid osseous dysplasia should be considered in the differential diagnosis.

Laboratory Aids

Serum calcium, phosphorous, and acid phosphatase are within normal limits. Alkaline phosphatase is generally markedly elevated, with values as high as 250 Bodansky units, especially during the osteoblastic phase of the disease. Urinalysis will demonstrate elevated values of hydroxyproline, which originates from destruction of bone collagen.

Treatment

The treatment is in the hands of a physician specialized in bone disorders. It consists essentially of massive doses of fluoride and magnesium with careful control of the patient in order to avoid bone marrow depletion. The disease is controlled with this therapy, but the condition is not eradicated.

Papillary Hyperplasia of the Palate (3D46)

This condition, also known as palatal papillomatosis, is an inflammatory nodular hyperplasia of the palate of unknown cause.

Clinical Features

Multiple, red, edematous, pebbly nodules appear on the hard palate medially, sometimes also involving the edematous alveolus. Individual papillae are about 1 mm in diameter. The patients are generally denture wearers, although some are not. The lesions often conform to relief chambers and other anatomic variations of the denture base. The condition persists and becomes more fibrous.

Differential Diagnosis (see p. 38)

Denture sore mouth, which can coexist with this condition, is the important discrimination to be made. The papules of nicotine stomatitis on the hard palate are seen around the orifices of the minor salivary glands.

Laboratory Aids

Histologically the lesion comprises multiple minute inflammatory polyps with marked pseudoepitheliomatous change. This has on occasion been misinterpreted as carcinoma, but there is general agreement that this is not a premalignant condition.

Treatment

Removal of the denture at night and use of tissue conditioner resolves the lesion in the early inflammatory stages. When fibrosis has occurred, surgical stripping is required.

Papilloma (3C26)

This growth is a benign neoplasm of epithelium of unknown etiology. It develops as hyperplastic, fingerlike projections of the epithelium each with a central core of fibrovascular stroma.

Clinical Features

Papilloma is usually a single, but occasionally multiple, small (up to 1 cm in diameter), pinkish white, exophytic, nodular or papular excrescence, most commonly found on the gingiva, the tongue, or the palatal mucosa. The lesion is painless and entirely benign in its behavior, remaining relatively small for long periods of time. Hyperkeratinization of the papilloma may give it a spiky texture and permit superadded infection with bacteria and fungi.

Differential Diagnosis (see p. 37)

Condyloma acuminatum (venereal warts) must be considered in the differential diagnosis because they are known to occur intraorally. The common wart rarely, if ever, occurs in the mouth. Multiple papillomas are also seen in focal dermal hypoplasia syndrome.

Laboratory Aids

Biopsy will demonstrate the nature of the lesion.

Treatment

Surgical excision is the treatment of choice.

Papillon-Lefèvre Syndrome (3A9, 3A10, and 3A11)

Papillon-Lefèvre syndrome, also known as hyperkeratosis palmoplantaris and periodontoclasia in childhood, consists of hyperkeratosis of the palms and soles and premature destruction of the periodontal ligament of both deciduous and permanent dentitions, with subsequent loss of teeth. The condition is inherited as an autosomal recessive.

Clinical Features

After normal eruption of the deciduous teeth, and concurrent with the initial appearance of the palmar and plantar hyperkeratosis, the gingiva becomes red, swollen, and boggy, and bleeds easily. Severe halitosis is noted. When the last primary molars complete eruption, destruction of the periodontal ligament begins, leading to the formation of deep periodontal pockets that exude pus upon pressure. Roentgenograms show a marked destruction of the supporting alveolar bone. The complete dentition becomes mobile, and by the age of 4 or 5 the child sheds all the teeth in approximately the same sequence in which they erupted. After the primary teeth are lost, gingival inflammation subsides and the oral cavity resumes its normal appearance, the patient being completely edentulous. The process is repeated in essentially the same manner for the permanent dentition. The patient generally becomes totally edentulous by the age of 15. After all permanent teeth are lost, the gingiva resumes its normal appearance. Dentures are tolerated well.

Hyperkeratosis palmoplantaris generally precedes periodontal involvement of the primary dentition. The palms usually present a well-demarcated, red, scaly hyperkeratosis extending to the margins and over the thenar eminences. The soles are involved to a greater degree, the process frequently spilling over the edges and onto the Achilles tendon. Occasionally, tibial tuberosities, external malleoli, and dorsum of finger and toe joints present hyperkeratotic plaques. The degree of hyperkeratosis increases in severity coincidentally with the acute periodontal manifestations. Fetid hyperhidrosis, especially of the feet, is frequent. Palmoplantar hyperkeratosis persists throughout life.

Differential Diagnosis (see p. 35)

All other forms of keratosis palmoplantaris, pachyonychia congenita, and conditions associated with premature loss of teeth in childhood, such as cyclic neutropenia, histiocytosis X, and idiopathic periodontosis, should be considered.

Laboratory Aids

None known.

Treatment

All therapeutic attempts to save the teeth, to date, have been unsuccessful. Maintenance of oral hygiene, to prevent superimposed infection, and palliative medication, to control pain, are recommended. After the teeth are exfoliated, patients will tolerate full-mouth dentures well. These should be changed according to the growth of the patient. The third molars are generally extracted immediately after eruption in order to prevent them from interfering with the dentures.

Parotid Gland Cyst (1E51)

Cysts arising from salivary gland tissue are rare and, when they do occur, are predominantly in the parotid. More common are branchial lymphoepithelial cysts (branchial cleft cyst), which occur within lymph nodes in a similar position (1E53).

Clinical Features

The cyst presents as a painless, single, fluctuant, well-circumscribed mass just above the angle of the mandible. The cyst can vary in size and occasionally may enlarge progressively.

Differential Diagnosis (see p. 11)

Lymph nodal pathology as well as neoplastic pathology of the parotid gland should be considered. Lateral cysts of the neck, such as branchial cleft cyst, must be included in the differential diagnosis.

Laboratory Aids

None.

Treatment

Surgical excision is the treatment of choice.

Parotitis, Acute (1E50)

This condition is an acute pyogenic infection of the parotid gland that occurs usually by a retrograde infection with staphylococci or streptococci. The majority of affected patients have a reduced salivary flow owing to fever, debility, or major surgery.

Clinical Features

The condition frequently manifests as a bilateral, firm swelling of both parotids that is accompanied by pain, redness, locally increased temperature, and discharge of pus from the orifice of the parotid duct. Elderly persons are more commonly affected. If left untreated, this parotitis can progress to a general infection with spread of the pus through tissue spaces.

Differential Diagnosis (see p. 11)

Other forms of parotid inflammatory pathology could be considered.

Laboratory Aids

Pus milked from Stensen's duct should be cultured for identification of the organism and for its antibiotic sensitivity.

Treatment

Antibiotic therapy is indicated. Surgical drainage should be employed in the event of a fluctuant abscess of the parotid.

Pemphigus Vulgaris (3B19)

Pemphigus vulgaris is an autoimmune disorder characterized by suprabasilar acantholysis within the epithelium of the skin and mucous membranes.

Clinical Features

Pemphigus vulgaris is generally seen in patients between 40 and 60 years of age, affecting both sexes equally. Essentially all patients with pemphigus vulgaris have oral manifestations, and in more than 50% of affected patients the initial manifestations are intraoral, sometimes preceding the skin changes by 2 years or more. The disease starts with the appearance of bullae of various sizes. Any area of the oral cavity can be affected. The intraoral bullae are generally of very short duration, rarely lasting more than a few hours. The bullae are tensive and round, and pressure on them causes lateral extension of the fluid into the apparently normal surrounding tissue because of acantholysis (Asboe-Hansen's sign). If either adjacent normal skin or mucous membrane is rubbed, the superficial layers will slough and/or new bullae may form (Nikolsky's sign). Skin bullae rupture easily and crust. Rupture of the oral bullae results in extensive ulceration with ragged margins and peripheral, whitish yellow sloughing of epithelium. Oral lesions are accompanied by minor bleeding and marked pain.

Denuded skin and mucous membrane lesions are painful and may become secondarily infected. Serious involvement of the oral mucosa makes ingestion of food difficult. Marked salivation is always present. When the skin is extensively involved, toxicity occurs. Anemia, hypoalbuminemia, serum electrolyte disturbances, and increased sedimentation rate are common findings in advanced pemphigus vulgaris.

After a somewhat insidious onset, the disease may progress rapidly in some patients, with a plethora of new bullae. Without treatment, pemphigus vulgaris progresses to a fatal outcome. In some patients the disease advances more slowly, with spontaneous remissions and exacerbations. Death usually results from cachexia toxicity or bacterial infection.

Differential Diagnosis (see p. 36)

All vesiculobullous and ulcerative diseases should be considered.

Laboratory Aids

Biopsy reveals acantholysis with intraepithelial bulla formation just above the basal cell layer. Cytologic smears of the base of an intraoral bulla will demonstrate the presence of detached acantholytic epithelial cells, which are characterized by enlarged hyperchromatic nuclei. These cells are known as Tzanck's cells. Antibodies against the epithelial cell membrane in pemphigus can be found both tissue-bound at the level of the spinous cell membrane and circulating in the blood of patients with active disease. Direct or indirect immunofluorescent procedures will demonstrate binding of IgG and complement to the cell membrane of the spinous epithelial layer. This finding is highly specific for all types of pemphigus. With the direct procedure, this reaction is noted in all pemphigus lesions and also in adjacent, clinically nonaffected skin or mucosal epithelium.

Treatment

Patients are generally referred to the dermatologist for treatment. Initial therapy consists of large doses of corticosteroids and antibiotics. The former induces remission of the lesion, and the latter controls secondary infection. Once remission is obtained, the patient is kept on maintenance doses of corticosteroids. The steroid therapy is used to arrest the abnormal immune reaction, but it does not actually effect a permanent cure for the disease.

Periapical Abscess (3D54; 4A11 and 4A12; 4E50 and 4E51; 4E58 and 4E59)

Acute periapical abscesses occur as the result of virulent pathogens and their products egressing from the nonvital root canal. The pus takes the line of least resistance through the alveolar plate to produce a subperiosteal abscess.

Clinical Features

Acute periapical abscess is accompanied by bone pain and the tooth is tender to touch because of concomitant acute periodontitis. Severe pain persists until the pus goes beyond the confines of the bone. A truly acute periapical abscess is not usually discernible in a radiograph. A subperiosteal abscess is identifiable as a fluctuant, sessile, well-defined mass adjacent to bone. The overlying tissues may be normal in color or may be acutely inflamed or discolored with blood pigment (as in 3E54). The abscess is often accompanied by an acute inflammatory edema of the surrounding facial or oral tissues. Drainage of the pus is usually effected by spontaneous rupture of the abscess, by surgical incision and drainage, or by extraction of the offending tooth. Drainage may resolve to a sinus opening. On occasion, rupture of the abscess may be accompanied by loss of gingival tissue and bone (as in 4E50 and 4E51). Periapical abscesses of deciduous molar teeth are frequently discharged through the periodontal ligament (as in 4A11 and 4A12). When drainage is established, rapid relief of the symptoms is experienced. Very rarely a dental abscess may spread to involve deeper tissue planes or cerebral sinuses.

Differential Diagnosis (see pp. 38, 47, 49, 50)

The clinical presentation is quite characteristic or indicative of the process. Nevertheless, other periapical lesions, such as cyst, might be considered. Rarely granulomatous inflammations will develop in that location.

Laboratory Aids

Pus from dental abscesses should be smeared and cultured in the event that excision and drainage does not completely resolve the lesion.

Treatment

Drainage of a periapical abscess can sometimes be effected by opening into the pulp chamber. Antibiotics may be prescribed but occasionally are ineffectual due to the inability of the antibiotic to penetrate the necrotic pus. Subperiosteal abscesses should be incised and drained and the offending tooth treated endodontically or extracted if endodontic treatment is not possible.

Periapical Cemental Dysplasia (5D43)

This condition is an aberration of periapical connective tissue in which a fibroblastic stroma is gradually replaced by cementumlike calcified tissue. The cause is unknown. The teeth remain vital.

Clinical Features

Multiple poorly defined periapical radiolucencies are found most commonly on the lower incisor, cuspid, and premolar teeth. This is the first, or osteolytic, stage of the process and resembles the periapical radiolucency of a periapical granuloma. In the subsequent stage, the lesion develops radiopaque flecks and more calcified material is laid down. In the final, inactive, phase the lesion presents as a periapical radiopacity resembling condensing osteitis. The lesion is painless. The teeth respond positively to vitality tests. There may be, however, a suggestion of traumatic occlusion. The condition appears to have a predilection for the lower incisor teeth of women. The lesion grows to a certain size and stops and matures with no complications.

Differential Diagnosis (see p. 61)

This lesion is to be discriminated from the true cementoma, a benign neoplasm of cementum that continues to grow steadily by peripheral extension. It is also discriminated from sclerosing or condensing osteitis by the lack of pulpal involvement. It is essential to differentiate the early osteolytic stage from periapical granuloma or cyst. Autosomal familial cemental dysplasia should also be considered as well as fibroosseous dysplasia.

Laboratory Aids

Pulp vitality tests are essential.

Treatment

Regular radiographic follow-up is indicated. No surgery is indicated unless the behavior of the lesion does not conform to the picture given here or clinical bone expansion is found.

Periapical Granuloma (1D45; 4B18 and 4B19; 4D41, 4D42, and 4D43; 4E57; 5D42)

Pulpal necrosis and gangrene are generally accompanied by some reaction at the tooth's apex. The most common of these is the periapical granuloma, which is a focal collection of chronic inflammatory cells surrounded by a fibrous tissue capsule. The immune reaction so mounted prevents the spread of infection beyond the root canal.

Clinical Features

The lesion is discernible on a periapical radiograph as an interruption of the lamina dura in the apical one-third of the tooth. The surrounding radiolucency of approximately 1 cm in diameter is either circular or pear shaped. The lesion may merge imperceptibly with the surrounding normal trabeculae or may be fairly well defined by a radiopaque margin. Destruction of the juxtacortical bone is necessary for the lesion to be seen on X ray. The lesion is generally painless but may be accompanied by a dull ache. The lesion is usually indolent and may last relatively unaltered for years; however, within the granuloma there is usually some epithelial proliferation derived from the cell rests of Malassez that eventually undergo cystic degeneration. The cyst may enlarge to encroach upon fairly large areas of mandible or maxilla. However, at an early stage, a periapical granuloma and a periapical dental cyst are one and the same pathologic process, and the two are indistinguishable radiographically. Pyogenic inflammation from either the granuloma or cyst may track through bone and soft tissue to open as a sinus in the oral mucosa or on the face.

Differential Diagnosis (see pp. 11, 48, 49, 50, 61)

Radiographically and according to the location, one should consider an early phase of periapical cemental dysplasia. Multiple periapical radiolucencies are seen in vitamin D-resistant rickets. Brown tumors of hyperparathyroidism could imitate periapical lesions.

Laboratory Aids

None, but biopsy should always be performed on these lesions if they are surgically removed.

Treatment

The lesion, in the majority of cases, regresses with effective root canal treatment.

Pericoronitis (2B15; 3B23)

Pericoronitis is an inflammation of the operculum, that is a flap of gingiva overlying an unerupted tooth, generally a mandibular third molar. It is formed as an ulceration of the epithelium directly overlying the crown of the unerupted tooth, which is in contact with bacterial contamination. Secondary trauma from the maxillary third molar may exacerbate the inflammation.

Clinical Features

A painful, swollen operculum overlying an impacted tooth may be accompanied by trismus and lymphadenitis. Infection of the pericoronal flap may be accompanied by fever and malaise. Progress to a pericoronal abscess may result in a fluctuant swelling, cellulitis, and tracking of pus through cervical tissue spaces. Rarely, cavernous sinus thrombophlebitis may ensue.

Differential Diagnosis (see p. 22, 36)

A similar condition may arise from primary herpetic infection of the gingiva.

Laboratory Aids

None.

Treatment

Hot saline mouth washes will reduce the inflammation. If, however, trismus and other general signs and symptoms are present, antibiotics should be prescribed. Operative procedures are contraindicated in the presence of acute pericoronitis.

Peutz-Jeghers's Syndrome (1C29)

Peutz-Jeghers's syndrome, also known as intestinal polyposis II, is characterized by mucocutaneous melanotic pigmentation and gastrointestinal polyposis. The condition is inherited as an autosomal dominant with high penetrance.

Clinical Features

The typical finding is the presence, in more than 50% of affected persons, of discrete, brown to bluish black macules of the skin, chiefly around the oral, nasal, and orbital orifices. The pigmented macules are generally not more than a few millimeters in diameter, and they vary in number and degree of pigmentation especially with age. Occasionally macules occur on the dorsum of the nose and other facial skin areas. Pigmentation of the extremities, conjunctiva, and nasal mucosa can also be found, with the number of pigmented spots varying in different patients. The lips, especially the lower, and the oral mucosa are involved with pigmented macules in about 98% of patients; less frequently the gingiva and palate and rarely the oral floor and the tongue are affected. The oral melanotic spots are larger than those on the skin, up to 12 mm in diameter.

The most important component of the syndrome is the polyposis of the gastrointestinal tract. The polyps are hamartomas and the following sites, in order of frequency, are involved: jejunum, ileum, large bowel, rectum, stomach, duodenum, and appendix. Some patients have had polyps of the bladder, nose, cervix, and bronchi, but this is unusual. There is no substantial evidence that the polyps are premalignant. Granulosa cell tumors of the ovary are found in a high percentage of affected females.

Polyps may produce intussusception and occasionally lead to severe intestinal obstruction and death. The age of onset of intestinal complications cannot be precisely determined, but generally there is a history of gastrointestinal problems before the third decade of life.

The cutaneous pigmented macules tend to fade after puberty, but the intraoral pigmentation remains for life. The older the patient, the fewer the number of macules and the less the degree of pigmentation.

Differential Diagnosis (see p. 10)

Intestinal polyposis I (colonic polyposis), Gardner's syndrome, Addison's disease, Fabry's syndrome, and Albright's syndrome should be considered in the differential diagnosis.

Laboratory Aids

Roentgenographic survey of the gastrointestinal tract is helpful in establishing the diagnosis.

Treatment

None for the pigmented macules. Intussusception requires surgical intervention. Genetic counseling is indicated as in any other inherited condition.

Pleomorphic Adenoma (1E52; 3E53)

Pleomorphic adenoma (mixed tumor) is the most frequent benign tumor of salivary glands affecting both major and minor glands. Rarely, a malignant version is seen, and in reality this is a variant of salivary gland adenocarcinoma.

Clinical Features

The neoplasm presents as a single, painless, slow-growing, sessile lump. The overlying epithelium is usually not ulcerated, and blood vessels of the capsule can be seen crossing its surface. The parotid is the most common major salivary gland affected (as in 1E52). The tumor generally develops in the tail of the gland. The palatal glands are the most frequently affected intraoral minor glands (as in 3E53). There, the lesions develop in the posterolateral third of the junction of the soft and hard palates. The upper lip can also be the site of such tumors. Pleomorphic adenoma generally occurs in patients over 30 years of age, but cases in young adults and children are known to occur. There seems to be a slight predilection for females. The tumor is encapsulated (in a pseudocapsule), but neoplastic cells can migrate into the capsule and proliferate into cellular nests that give rise to small buddings or projections from the capsule. This phenomenon accounts for the great number of recurrences of this lesion, especially in those cases that have been improperly surgically removed. If untreated, the neoplasm can progressively reach remarkable size.

Differential Diagnosis (see pp. 12, 38)

Depending upon the location, one should consider other neoplasms or cysts of salivary glands, as well as granulomatous diseases or inflammatory pathology.

Laboratory Aids

Biopsy will demonstrate the nature of the lesion.

Treatment

Careful surgical dissection is the indicated treatment. If the tumors develop in the superficial parotid lobe, extreme care must be taken in order not to damage the facial nerve.

Pulp Necrosis, Traumatic (4D47 and 4D48; 5D48 and 4E49)

Traumatic necrosis of the pulp is generally due to thrombosis of the apical vessels, secondary to trauma to the area. The pulp undergoes aseptic infarction. The infarct may eventually become secondarily infected.

Necrosis of the pulp can also be found under unlined silicate restorations (4D42 and 4D43). High acid content of silicate cements has traditionally been implicated with the death of the pulp. However, recent findings call this theory into question. First, the amount of free acid is not thought sufficient to cause the death of the pulp, and, second, silicate cement is found to have no bacteriocidal capacity, in contrast to the zinc phosphate cement normally used as a lining material. Consequently, it is now suggested that the loss of tooth vitality associated with unlined silicate restorations is due to bacterial infection.

Clinical Features

After the pain of the trauma and subsequent inflammation have resolved, the necrosis is painless. The tooth, however, will lose its translucency and the dentin may become stained brown or black by hematogenous pigment. The tooth will respond negatively to vitality tests. On opening into the pulp chamber only dry necrotic material may be found. Infection of the necrotic material may take weeks, months, or even years, after which time radiographic evidence of a periaptical granuloma may be apparent. The patient may have symptoms of dull ache or pain. The pulp chamber may contain gangrenous and foul-smelling material.

Periapical abscess and cellulitis may supervene, or a periapical sinus may be established to the buccal mucosa (as in 4D47).

Traumatic pulp necrosis can be secondary to gold foil condensation (as in 4E48 and 4E59). The action of the automatic mallet in condensing gold foil against the dentinal walls of the cavity produces microtrauma to the pulp and the periapical vessels, and can result in traumatic pulp necrosis. Partial or total displacement of teeth and intrusion or extrusion of teeth as a result of trauma may also produce pulp necrosis. The attempt to maintain teeth after such trauma is also accompanied, to some extent, by external resorption of the root (as in 5E49).

Differential Diagnosis (see pp. 49, 61)

Questioning of the patient to ascertain the cause of the necrosis is mandatory.

Laboratory Aids

None.

Treatment

Endodontic therapy is indicated.

Pulp Stones (4C35)

Calcific masses of various size and shape may occur within the pulp chamber, apparently under physiologic conditions. Calcification is thought to arise in blood vessel walls and to increase with age. Increased numbers are also apparent in relationship to carious cavities.

Clinical Features

The condition is usually an incidental finding on radiographs, where the pulp stones present as diffuse or fairly regular calcifications of the pulp chamber and root canals. There is no evidence that pulp stones are responsible for dental pain. The only potential complication is an obstruction to root canal therapy.

Differential Diagnosis (see p. 49)

Obliteration of pulp chambers can be seen in other disorders, such as dentinal dysplasia and dentinogenesis imperfecta. In both of these conditions tooth shape and generality of the involvement will establish the diagnosis.

Laboratory Aids

None.

Treatment

None.

Pulpitis, Chronic Hyperplastic (4E49)

Chronic hyperplastic pulpitis is an inflammatory hyperplasia of the dental pulp (pulp polyp), a relatively rare sequel of carious destruction of the tooth crown and exposure of the tooth pulp in the teeth of children and young adults with large apical foramina and good blood supply. The lesion may become secondarily epithelialized.

Clinical Features

This lesion presents as a single polypoid mass of reddish pink granulation tissue protruding from the pulp chamber of heavily carious deciduous molars or first permanent molars in children and young adults. The lesion is surprisingly painless. The pulp in the root canals is vital, and periapical involvement is absent. The lesion grows very slowly and may remain static over months or even years. If traumatized during mastication, it may be painful and bleed.

Differential Diagnosis (see p. 49)

Inflammatory hyperplasia originating in the gingiva or periodontal ligament and extending into the tooth needs to be considered.

Laboratory Aids

None.

Treatment

The tooth is generally extracted, though endodontic therapy may be contemplated in first permanent molars.

Pyogenic Granuloma (3C29; 3C31; 3C33)

Pyogenic granuloma is an exuberant overgrowth of neocapillaries and fibrous connective tissue caused by minor mechanical or microbial plaque irritation. These growths are apparently prone to occur in pregnant women, in women taking oral contraceptives simulating pregnancy, and, rarely, in patients taking diphenylhydantoin sodium. Tooth sockets provide a favorable environment.

Clinical Features

This condition generally manifests as a painless, easily bleeding, ulcerated, red, polypoid mass with a broad base, usually located on the marginal gingiva. It can also be found on the lips, the tongue, the buccal mucosa, the palate, the vestibule, and even the alveolar mucosa of edentulous patients. Because of hormonal influences, the lesion is most common in young adult females. The lesion initially grows fairly rapidly to attain a diameter of a few millimeters or sometimes 2 cm or more. It then tends to mature to a more fibrous and less ulcerated form and may finally become a dense peripheral fibrous gingival hyperplasia (as in 3C30). This maturation process is particularly marked postpartum in "pregnancy tumors." Radiographically, there may be a slight resorption of interdental septal bone.

Differential Diagnosis (see p. 37)

Periapical fibrous hyperplasia and peripheral giant cell granuloma should be considered. Antral prolapse should be investigated if the lesion is in a maxillary tooth socket.

Laboratory Aids

Biopsy will reveal marked capillary proliferation and superimposed inflammatory infiltrate.

Treatment

Surgical excision is the treatment of choice. In its highly vascular stage the lesion is prone to recur with an alarmingly rapid growth. More fibrous lesions are less likely to recur. It is better to delay the removal of pregnancy tumors until after delivery. Plaque control is indicated.

Radicular Cyst (4D41; 4E55) and Residual Dental Cyst (5D39)

The periapical odontogenic cyst is an inflammatory cyst derived from the epithelial rests of Malassez. It arises at the apex of a tooth whose pulp is destroyed by necrosis or gangrene. Persistence of the cyst after tooth extraction is rare, but when it does occur it is known as a residual cyst. The epithelial rest undergoes proliferation and subsequent cystic degeneration in the center of a previous periapical granuloma.

Clinical Features

This cyst presents as a sessile swelling of different sizes, within bone or involving soft tissue, always associated with decayed teeth or teeth with necrotic pulp of various etiologies. The peripheral bone may become so thinned as to produce a crackling on palpation. The cyst, when in the maxilla, may extend to involve the antrum. Nodes are not involved unless the cyst is secondarily infected. Radiographically the lesion is a radiolucency of varying size surrounding the apex of a nonvital tooth or tooth root. The cyst is generally slow growing and may be present for several years without causing symptoms. Prognosis is usually excellent, although an occasional case results in fracture of the jaw. A handful of cases have been reported in which the cystic epithelial lining has undergone transformation into a squamous cell carcinoma; in those cases, additional symptoms of pain or lack of sensation in involved nerves may be apparent. The residual dental cyst is a periapical cyst that remains or has been accidentally left behind after tooth extraction. The cyst presents as a radiolucency within bone, of variable size and with perfectly delineated borders. It is generally asymptomatic.

Differential Diagnosis (see pp. 49, 50, 61)

Periapical granuloma is the prime consideration, but unfortunately this differentiation can only be established under the microscope. Early cementomas, during the radiolucent phase, should be considered if the lesion occurs in the anterior mandibular teeth. Brown tumors of hyperparathyroidism can also mimic periapical pathology. Depending on the location, the residual dental cyst needs to be differentiated from the static bone cyst and the nasopalatine cyst.

Laboratory Aids

Biopsy of any periapical or residual lesion should be a routine procedure.

Treatment

Many periapical cysts, radiologically indistinguishable from periapical granulomas, are effectively treated by endodontic therapy. Large cysts are normally enucleated, however, in very extensive lesions; marsupialization of the cyst wall to the oral mucosa may effect obliteration. The residual cyst is treated with surgical excision or, if large, is marsupialized.

Ranula (1E56; 2C31)

A ranula is a large mucocele associated with the sublingual and occasionally with the submandibular duct system in the floor of the mouth. Its etiology is identical to that of the mucocele; that is, it results from an injury to or a rupture of the salivary duct system in the affected area. Some authors believe that it is produced by a ductal aneurysm.

Clinical Features

Ranula is a rare condition that develops very slowly. It is generally deeply located. Therefore, the overlying oral mucosa is usually normal in color. The condition is unilateral, and bimanual palpation demonstrates fluctuation. The floor of the mouth in the affected side demonstrates the tumorlike mass. Large ranulas may also protrude into the neck. Some cases of superficial lesions have been described.

Differential Diagnosis (see pp. 12, 23)

Intraorally, epidermoid and dermoid cysts should be considerd, as well as neoplastic pathology of the sublingual and submandibular salivary glands. Extraorally, the differential diagnosis will include a large number of lesions manifested as neck masses.

Laboratory Aids

Sialography can be used to demonstrate the glandular blockage.

Treatment

Surgical excision is the treatment of choice. Large ranulas are surgically treated with marsupialization.

Regional Enteritis (2A10)

Regional enteritis, also known as Crohn's disease, is an inflammatory disease of the ileum of suspected autoimmune pathogenesis; it can also affect any part of the gastrointestinal tract, including the mouth and the anus.

Clinical Features

Several oral manifestations have been described in patients with the disease, such as red granular lesions ("cobblestoning"), linear ulcerations, hypertrophic tags, erythema migrans of most mucosal surfaces, edema of the lips, and granulomatous cheilitis. The lesions are annoyingly painful and may cause dysphagia. They predominate in patients with active disease, and occasionally oral manifestations may appear before the systemic symptoms. Some oral lesions persist for 10 years or longer. Diffuse scarring of the oral mucosa may result. Pharyngeal and laryngeal spread of the condition can also occur.

Differential Diagnosis (see p. 22)

Aphthous ulceration, Behçet's disease, sarcoidosis, cheilitis glandularis apostematosa, and Melkersson-Rosenthal's syndrome should be considered.

Laboratory Aids

Low serum albumin and raised seromucoid levels are indicative of active disease. Salivary IgA secretion rate will be lower than normal. Biopsy will show abnormal focal collections of plasma cells and lymphocytes. Perivascular mononuclear cell infiltrates, similar to the gastrointestinal lesions, will be found in the lamina propria of the oral mucosa. Noncaseating sarcoidlike giant cell granulomas may also be found.

Treatment

Topical corticosteroids are often beneficial. Surgery for the gastrointestinal lesions may alleviate the oral lesions.

Resorption of Teeth (4B13; 4D39; 5D48 and 5E49)

Osteoclasts may resorb enamel, dentin, or cementum in a variety of pathological situations.

Clinical Features

Resorption of teeth takes several forms. External resorption of enamel may take place in unerupted teeth when the protective effect of the reduced enamel epithelium is lost. External resorption of the radicular dentin occurs when the protective effect of the cementum is lost by trauma or periodontal disease. Internal resorption of dentin from the pulpal aspect is thought to arise from a local vascular abnormality and is less common than external resorption.

External resorption of unerupted teeth (as in 4D39) is seen as a progressive loss of the coronal enamel and dentin; it gradually extends to encompass the root and pulp chamber. As the resorbed dental tissue is removed it is replaced by bone. Since this process takes many years, it tends to be found in older individuals, and ankylosis may complicate an attempt to remove the tooth. Resorption of the roots of erupted teeth is the more common type of external resorption. It occurs in teeth damaged by trauma or by excessive orthodontic tooth movement and in reimplanted teeth. Degrees of periapical resorption are seen associated with periapical granulomas and cysts, and idiopathic root resorption has also been described. Granulation tissue is frequently found within the periodontium occupying the cavity, and secondary caries may intervene.

Internal resorption is found radiographically as a round or oval central radiolucent area, generally in the middle one-third of the tooth. Symptoms are usually absent, though a dull, pulsating pain may occasionally be found in advanced resorption. Deep palatal pits and fissures of the cingulum may be present. Periapical radiolucency should be looked for. Laterally, the resorption may perforate and, if in the crown, will show as a pink spot.

Differential Diagnosis (see pp. 47, 49, 61, 62)

Idiopathic root resorption is also seen in malignant and benign tumors of the maxilla and mandible. Internal tooth resorption in unerupted teeth is seen in some forms of ectodermal dysplasia.

Laboratory Aids

None.

Treatment

Endodontic therapy may be attempted with true internal resorption. Since the latter is extremely rare, the possible point of ingress of external resorption should be sought for diligently.

Sclerosing Osteitis (4D47 and 4D48; 5C27; 5C28; 5C30)

This condition, also known as condensing osteitis, is a focal increase in density of bone as a response to chronic inflammation around the apices of chronically inflamed or nonvital teeth.

Clinical Features

The lesion presents as a radiopacity of varying size, shape, and contour. The lesions are generally not well defined. The periodontal membrane's space is seen to enter the lesion, but the lamina dura may be seen to have lost its integrity, distinguishing sclerosing oseitis from hypercementosis, where the periodontal membrane's space and the lamina dura surround the lesions (as in 5C29). Acute symptoms such as pain, swelling and drainage, and lymphadenitis are absent, though some degree of periapical sclerosis may be seen associated with a dental sinus (as in 4D48). After root canal therapy or extraction of the tooth, the sclerosis may not necessarily disappear (as in 5C27).

Differential Diagnosis (see pp. 49, 60)

Depending upon the location, periapical cemental dysplasia and benign cementoblastoma need to be considered in the differential diagnosis.

Laboratory Aids

Pulp vitality tests may be equivocal, since sclerosing osteitis may occur in teeth that have one nonvital root canal and two vital root canals.

Treatment

Root canal therapy is the indicated treatment.

Sialadenitis (1E57)

Sialadenitis is a chronic, nonspecific inflammation of salivary glands usually due to obstruction by a sialolith.

Clinical Features

The submandibular gland is most commonly affected by this recurrent, generally painless swelling. The enlargement is unilateral, and palpation demonstrates a brawny swelling. Intraoral examination reveals diminished or absent salivary flow in the affected side. Asymmetry of the upper neck is evident on facial examination. By way of complication, dilations of the ducts (sialectasis) and fibrosis of the acinar portion of the gland may occur.

Differential Diagnosis (see p. 12)

Lymph node pathology, neck cysts, and neoplastic pathology of salivary glands should be considered.

Laboratory Aids

Retrograde sialography with the injection of radiopaque materials through the duct may be of assistance in delineating sialectases.

Treatment

Removal of the sialolith or, in long-standing cases, surgical removal of the affected gland are indicated.

Sialolithiasis (1E57; 2C26; 2C29 and 2C30)

Sialolithiasis refers to the formation of a calcified mass within the duct of a major or minor salivary gland, thought to be due to the precipitation of calcium salts from the saliva upon desquamated epithelial cells, bacteria or salivary proteins.

Clinical Features

The sialolith (or calculus) is usually a single ellipsoid mass, approximately 1 cm at its largest dimension, that can be palpated in the duct as a hard mass. If it is near the ductal orifice, it may show through the overlying epithelium as a yellowish mass (as in 2C26). Sialoliths occur most commonly in the submandibular glands. The parotid is the next most commonly affected gland, and the sublingual is less commonly affected. Sialoliths of minor salivary glands (as in 2C26) are relatively uncommon. Blockage of the duct is accompanied by pain and rapid swelling (as in 1E57), particularly at mealtime. Blockage and retrograde infection may result in sialadenitis. Radiographically the lesion presents as a radiopacity within the soft tissues, with a concentric pattern of lamellated calcification as in (2C30).

Differential Diagnosis (see pp. 12, 23)

The clinical diagnosis is not a difficult one; nevertheless, other inflammatory pathology of salivary glands should be considered in the differential diagnosis.

Laboratory Aids

None.

Treatment

Sialoliths near the orifices of the ducts may be expressed by manipulation. Deeper involvement with sialadenitis may require surgical removal of the gland.

Silver Pigmentation (3D37)

Silver pigmentation, or argyria, is a skin or mucosal pigmentation caused by silver intoxication. A history may be elicited of self-medication for several years with nasal drops containing silver salts.

Clinical Features

Clinically, silver pigmentation manifests as a diffuse slate-blue pigmentation of the skin usually found on areas exposed to the sun. Intraoral pigmentation of the palatal mucosa may be related to nasal inhalation, the palate having a similar color to that seen on the skin.

Impairment of hearing and equilibrium due to damage to the VIII cranial nerve pair have been reported in silver intoxication.

Differential Diagnosis (see p. 37)

The blue nevus and lentigo maligna melanoma, which can occur on the palatal mucosa, should be ruled out by biopsy.

Laboratory Aids

Silver may be demonstrated histologically in the dermis.

Treatment

Medication should be stopped. Rapid postural change in and out of the dental chair should be avoided in cases of disequilibrium.

Squamous Cell Carcinoma (1C36; 1D40; 1D48; 2A8; 2B22; 2B23; 2C34; 2D38; 2D41; 3B24; 3C25; 3E51; 4E56)

Squamous cell carcinoma is a malignant neoplasm of epithelium that makes up more than 90% of all the malignant neoplasms occurring in the oral cavity. Oral carcinoma represents between 4% and 8% of all cancers diagnosed annually in the United States, that is, about 26,000 cases yearly. Two-thirds of the cases are fatal, with a mortality rate in the United States of from 5 to 10 per 100,000 persons. Approximately 90% of oral cancer patients are over 45 years of age, with a mean age of 60 years. When all intraoral locations are grouped, there is a male-to-female ratio of 2 to 1.

In this country, the incidence figures vary with geographic location not only for oral site but also for male-to-female ratio. This variation is partially due to tobacco habits (e.g., tobacco chewing is more common in the southeastern United States than elsewhere in the country). Variations in the incidence of oral cancers are also seen in different countries. A high frequency is observed in India and Southeast Asia, where it represents almost 50% of all cancers. This may be due to such habits as betel nut chewing and reverse smoking.

There is a relationship between the development of intraoral carcinoma and tobacco usage in its different forms, heavy intake of alcohol, and possibly tertiary syphilis. Surveys have shown that about 90% of patients with oral carcinoma are heavy smokers, and 75% admit heavy consumption of alcohol. The incidence of hepatic cirrhosis in patients with oral squamous cell carcinoma in the same group of patients has been estimated at 45%.

Clinical Features

Clinically, oral squamous cell carcinoma varies greatly. Early lesions can present as a white patch with an inconspicuous rough surface, as a slightly erythematous area, or even as a small exophytic growth. Any of the three may be associated with ulceration. One of the frequent early manifestations is the association of areas of rough whitening with erythematous areas.

Advanced lesions generally correspond to any one or a combination of ulcerative, exophytic, or verrucous varieties. Regardless of the site of occurrence, any of the above most usually presents a broad base that is hard on palpation. Pain is almost always absent in the initial stages, with the exception of lingual carcinoma. The tumor grows rapidly, and necrosis with subsequent ulceration is a frequent complication. The verrucous variety is composed of multiple papillary projections that generally extend superficially. Ulceration is rare in this form, which is considered an independent entity with a much more favorable prognosis. Further data for oral squamous cell carcinoma is presented in Table 3.

Table 3. Incidence of Oral Squamous Cell Carcinoma

Location	Percentage of Incidence	Male-to-Female Ratio	Age Range	Most Frequent Site	Percentage Showing Metastasis at Admission	Percentage Having 5-Year Survival
Lip	25-30 (95% lower lip)	14 to 1	50-70	Vermilion border	18	80-90
Tongue	25-30	4 to 1	60-80	Lateral border	40	35
Floor of mouth	10-15	5 to 1	50-60	Anterior floor	28	40-50
Gingiva and alveolar mucosa	5-10	4 to 1	60-80	Mandible	30	50
Buccal mucosa	5-10	4 to 1	Over 50	Left side	65	25

Differential Diagnosis (see pp. 10, 11, 22, 23, 24, 36, 38, 50)

A great variety of conditions can be considered in the differential diagnosis, depending on clinical appearance and location. Among the most frequent are white lesions (leukoplakia, lichen planus), traumatic ulceration, granulomatous diseases, and other neoplasms. Clinical signs to be kept in mind as quite indicative of a malignant neoplasm are induration, fixation to deeper structures, advanced age of the patient, and rapid growth of the lesion in a short period of time.

The Plummer-Vinson's syndrome has been associated with a high incidence of oral carcinoma. The condition is characterized by chronic iron deficiency and was most often observed in Scandinavian women. The oral mucosa becomes atrophic, and this seems to predispose to oral carcinoma. Now, the syndrome is seldom seen, due to better diet and vitamin B intake. Other syndromes may also be associated with oral squamous cell carcinoma, such as epidermolysis bullosa and xeroderma pigmentosum.

Laboratory Aids

Incisional biopsy will demonstrate the nature of the lesion.

Treatment

The treatment is in the hands of a specialized team of oncologists and depends on location, size, presence or absence of involved lymph nodes, and/or metastatic disease. Surgery, radiation therapy, chemotherapy, or a combination of these methods is employed in treating and controlling squamous cell carcinoma.

Sturge-Weber's Anomalad (1A8 and 1A9)

Sturge-Weber's anomalad, also known by the name of encephalofacial angiomatosis, is probably a consequence of the persistence of an intrauterine vascular plexus that develops around the cephalic portion of the neural tube. This structure should normally regress during the ninth to tenth week of development.

Clinical Features

The salient clinical finding is the presence of a superficial nevus flammeus, which is present in approximately 90% of affected patients. It generally extends from the forehead to the upper lip and occupies one-half of the face. Rarely, it may be bilateral, and in some instances it may also extend into the mandible. Intraorally, either superficial, flat, or hypertrophic angiomatous lesions can be found on the buccal mucosa and lips. The palate can also be affected, and, rarely, the tongue may be involved. Gingival lesions can present a similar appearance, sometimes mimicking hypertrophic fibromatosis. These lesions are well vascularized, and the danger of hemorrhage is always present. Associated findings include occasional delayed eruption of teeth on the affected side. Systemic findings include the presence of a unilateral angioma in the leptomeninges on the same side as the superficial angioma of the skin. Occasionally, calcification of the falx cerebri is observed. Approximately 30% of these patients exhibit some degree of mental deficiency. Seizures are observed in about 90% of affected individuals. All cases reported have been sporadic.

Differential Diagnosis (see p. 9)

The differential diagnosis should include Klippel-Trénaunay-Weber's syndrome. Other lesions, such as isolated superficial hemangioma, should be considered.

Laboratory Aids

Skull roentgenograms will show the presence of calcification, and electroencephalographic studies will demonstrate an unusual pattern.

Treatment

None.

Syphilis (1B13; 1C27; 1C35; 2D40; 2E52; 3E60; 4A10)

Syphilis is a chronic progressive disease produced by the spirochete *Treponema pallidum*.

Clinical Features

The primary stage of syphilis (as in 1C35) is characterized clinically as follows. After an incubation period of from 12 to 40 days, with 21 days being the average, a primary chancre develops at the site of inoculation. Multiple chancres may occur in some cases. Occasionally, the infection bypasses the primary stage and no chancre is observed. The chancre is a round to oval, brownish red, painless, ulcerated nodule with peripheral induration. Primary oral chancres are rare. When the chancre occurs on the lip, it is usually covered by a dark brown crust. Intraorally, the lesion may be covered with a grayish pseudomembrane. Pain may be a feature of intraoral lesions due to secondary infection. The chancre is an extremely infectious lesion because of its high spirochete content. Regional lymphadenopathy is always associated with the primary chancre, the involved lymph nodes being hard, movable, and painless.

The chancre heals without scarring within 2 to 4 weeks. Secondary infection of the chancre may prolong its course. If untreated, the disease progresses to the secondary stage.

The secondary stage (as in 1B13; 2D40) is heralded by mild fever, sore throat, lymphadenopathy, and a maculopapular eruption of the skin and oral mucosa 6 to 8 weeks after the appearance of the chancre. Intraorally, mucous patches — oval or irregular grayish white pseudomembranous lesions — are scattered on the buccal mucosa, the tongue, and the gingiva. Erythematous macules and maculopapular lesions without erosion may also occur on the oral mucosa, frequently on the palate. When papular lesions occur at the labial commissures, they frequently become fissured and are referred to as split papules. Oral lesions of secondary syphilis are also extremely infectious and represent a positive source of transmission.

The secondary stage of the disease is variable and may last for several weeks or as long as a year. Exacerbations of secondary syphilis may occur. As the secondary stage disappears, a latent period of variable duration occurs in which the patient is symptom free. At any time, however, tertiary syphilis may appear.

The tertiary lesions of syphilis (as in 2E52; 3E60) in the oral cavity consist of gummatous infiltration and diffuse syphilitic glossitis. Gummatous infiltration is most commonly observed at the midline of the palate. Gummatous involvement of the tongue may produce lingua lobulata. In interstitial glossitis, the papillae become markedly atrophic, producing the characteristic bald tongue. Shrinkage of involved tongue musculature may produce wrinkling of the dorsum. Gummatous infiltration may lead to marked irregularity of the oral tissues and perforation of the palate. Syphilitic glossitis predisposes to leukoplakia and is associated with squamous cell carcimona in 30% of the patients.

In congenital syphilis (as in 1C27; 4A10) mucocutaneous eruptions, rhinitis, and many other manifestations may be observed during the neonatal period. A mucopurulent discharge from the nose may excoriate the upper lip. Lesions at the labial commissures, which produce deep fissures, heal with radiating scars or rhagades. Gummatous destruction of nasal bones may produce saddle nose. In late congenital syphilis, Hutchinson's triad of interstitial keratitis, eighth cranial nerve involvement, and deformed central incisors may be observed in some patients. The three features of Hutchinson's triad are frequently not present in the same patient. Tooth anomalies are often absent in congenital syphilis. When they do occur, the permanent teeth are affected. Maxillary central incisors may be screwdriver shaped or notched along the incisal edge (Hutchinson's incisors). Mulberry molars may be noted in some patients. Permanent teeth may be generally hypoplastic; rarely, hypoplasia of deciduous teeth has been observed.

Differential Diagnosis (see pp. 9, 10, 24, 25, 39, 47)

A primary chancre may resemble squamous cell carcinoma. Intraoral lesions of secondary syphilis may resemble lichen planus or drug eruption. Gummatous infiltration may simulate carcinoma and a variety of granulomatous diseases. Atrophy of the tongue may be observed in vitamin deficiencies, in anemia, in long-standing lichen planus, and after antibiotic therapy.

Laboratory Aids

Dark-field examination may be effective for primary chancres of the lip. However, intraoral lesions are contaminated with normal oral flora such as *T. microdentium* and *T. macrodentium,* which are extremely difficult to differentiate from *T. pallidum*. Serologic tests such as complement fixation and flocculation tests are useful screening devices. Such tests may not be positive during the early evolution of the chancre but become positive shortly and are always positive during the secondary stage. False positive reactions may occur in collagen diseases or in any other disorder in which hypergammaglobulinemia is a feature. More specific tests for syphilis include the fluorescent treponemal antibody absorption (FTA-ABS) test and the *Treponema pallidum* immobilization (TPI) test, which represent the patient's immune status to the organism. Biopsy of chancres and gummatous lesions is occasionally necessary to rule out carcinoma.

Treatment

The treatment of syphilis is in the hands of the physician, and it essentially consists of adequate doses of antibiotics. Treatment is most effective during the primary period. The secondary and tertiary periods generally have a longer treatment. Positive serologic reactions are observed in the majority of patients even years after the completion of successful treatment.

Taurodontism (4D37)

Taurodontism refers to a tooth form characterized by an external block configuration. This condition is probably the result of a failure of epithelial root sheath to differentiate early and induce the normal root formation. In some families taurodontism is inherited as an autosomal dominant.

Clinical Features

The teeth, especially molars, are very large, with a square, block configuration. Radiographically the pulp chamber is very large, and the bifurcation or trifurcation of the molar teeth is apically placed. On radiograph this configuration gives the tooth the appearance of a pyramid, with a single root and a very small division at the apical area. Taurodontism is a racial trait, frequently observed among Eskimos and natives of Australia and Central America. Taurodont molars are also observed in the majority of patients with an extra X chromosome, including those with Klinefelter's syndrome or other variations on the number of X chromosomes. Taurodont teeth can also be associated with some other syndromes of very rare occurrence.

Differential Diagnosis (see p. 49)

In the case of males, the differential diagnosis should be established to rule out the possibility that the patient might be affected by Klinefelter's syndrome or any tetraploid XY syndromes.

Laboratory Aids

Radiographs will demonstrate the typical appearance of these teeth. No other aids are known.

Treatment

None.

Tetracycline Enamel Hypoplasia (4B24 and 4C25)

Administration of tetracycline during the period of tooth formation induces discoloration of the teeth being formed at that time. If the doses are large and prolonged, not only discoloration but also abnormal formation of enamel (i.e., enamel hypoplasia) is observed. Tetracycline and similar drugs have the capability of being deposited in calcified tissues during the process of calcification. Therefore, it has a marked affinity for bone, dentin, and enamel. Tetracycline is able to cross placental circulation; therefore, it will affect those teeth being formed during intrauterine development. Owing to the chronology of tooth formation the drug will have a time-dependent effect. Therefore, the exact time of administration of the drug can be easily determined by considering the teeth affected.

Clinical Features

The teeth affected by tetracycline will show a yellowish or brownish gray discoloration, but only in those areas formed during administration of the drug. With time, and especially by exposure of the teeth to sunlight, this discoloration will change to a marked brown color. If the teeth are exposed in a dark room to black light, they will fluoresce with a typical yellow color. The dentin is more heavily deposited with tetracycline than the enamel. In cases of high doses and prolonged administration of the drug, marked areas of hypoplasia will be seen, as in the case presented here.

Differential Diagnosis (see p. 48)

The differential diagnosis should include all conditions capable of producing generalized discoloration of teeth, such as erythroblastosis foetalis and porphyria. In advanced cases of enamel hypoplasia, amelogenesis imperfecta and dentinogenesis imperfecta should be considered in the differential diagnosis.

Laboratory Aids

As mentioned above, a black light is a great aid in the differential diagnosis, because teeth affected by tetracycline will react with a marked yellowish fluorescence (as in 4B25).

Treatment

Teeth can be capped for aesthetic and functional reasons. Capping facilitates mastication.

Thrombocytopenic Purpura (3D38)

Purpura is a clinical manifestation characterized by purple intramucosal or intradermal hemorrhages of various sizes. Therefore, purpura per se is not considered a disease but rather a clinical manifestation of a large number of blood disorders. Thrombocytopenic purpura, or thrombocytopenia, is characterized by a reduction in the number of circulating platelets. When the platelets are diminished in number, areas of local hemorrhage with consequent purpuric lesions will be observed. There are two different types of thrombocytopenic purpura. The primary type is thought to be of autoimmune etiology. The secondary type is produced by a great variety of etiologic agents including radiation, infection, metabolic disorders, hypothyroidism, and others. The two conditions have similar clinical manifestations.

Clinical Features

Purpuric lesions appear spontaneously on the skin and mucous membrane, and they vary in size from very small lesions to very large purple hematomalike ecchymoses. A tendency to bruise easily is evident in patients with thrombocytopenia. Bleeding from the nose or the gingiva is frequently found in these patients, and hemorrhage in the urinary and gastrointestinal tracts can also be observed. The majority of affected patients are below 30 years of age and there is no sex predilection. Frequent intraoral manifestations are gingival hemorrhage, which can be profuse, as well as purpuric lesions in the palate, as illustrated in the present case. Other mucous membranes can be similarly affected.

Differential Diagnosis (see p. 37)

The differential diagnosis of the intraoral lesions can include a great variety of blood disorders, including leukemia. In addition, purpuric lesions of the soft palate should include hematomas associated with vomiting efforts and hematomas associated with capillary fragility, sometimes induced by excessive intake of drugs such as aspirin. Purpuric lesions of the soft palate have been observed as a post fellatio consequence.

Laboratory Aids

The number of platelets in circulating blood of patients with this disorder is generally below 60,000 platelets per cubic millimeter. The bleeding time is prolonged, but the coagulation time is within normal limits.

Treatment

To date, no specific treatment is known for this condition. Thrombocytopenic purpura is known to regress by itself, and it is also known to recur. In severe cases, splenectomy is beneficial for these patients.

Thyroglossal Tract Cyst (1E58)

Thyroglossal tract cyst is a developmental abnormality that occurs due to cystic transformation of remnants of the epithelial tissue that gives rise to the thyroid gland. The thyroid gland begins developing at the base of the anterior portion of the tongue, exactly at the apex of the lingual V, as an invagination of the lingual epithelium. This invagination moves progressively downward in the center line of the neck until it reaches the final position that the thyroid gland should occupy. This invagination gives rise to an epithelial tract that normally should be reabsorbed. Occasionally, rests of this epithelium remain along the tract, and the cyst can occur at any point of this tract.

Clinical Features

The cyst can be observed at any point of the neck midline and occasionally has been observed intraorally at the base of the tongue or in the deep structures of the tongue. The most frequent location is the center of the neck, slightly above the thyroid gland. The cyst generally does not produce any clinical manifestation unless it becomes secondarily infected. Occasionally, it will protrude into the skin of the neck, and it may be accompanied by secondary inflammatory symptomatology.

Differential Diagnosis (see p. 12)

Other cysts of the neck, including epidermoid and dermoid cysts, should be considered in the differential diagnosis, as should tumors of the thyroid and/or parathyroid glands.

Laboratory Aids

None.

Treatment

Surgical elimination is the treatment of choice if the cyst is in a superficial location.

Tooth Stain, Exogenous (4C29; 4C30)

Exogenous tooth stain is produced by a great variety of chromogenic bacteria and is essentially found only in children.

Clinical Features

The color of the stain varies with the type of bacteria involved. Pigmentations in black, green and orange have been described. These pigments are deposited in the cervical one-third of both the buccal and lingual surfaces of the teeth. The stain is generally observed in youngsters between the ages of 6 and 14 years. Black stain tends to develop only in children who are caries free. Green and orange stain are associated with increased incidence of caries.

Differential Diagnosis (see p. 48)

The differential diagnosis should be established with reference to various types of stain, as well as dental plaque and early caries formation.

Laboratory Aids

None.

Treatment

Prophylaxis and treatment of caries when present are indicated.

Torus Mandibularis (3C34; 5D44)

Torus mandibularis is a bony exostosis of the mandible that is inherited as an autosomal dominant.

Clinical Features

This lesion can be unilateral, but it is mostly bilateral, occurring generally at the level of the premolar area in the lingual surface of the mandible. It can be a single lobule or a bilobulated area, variable in size. These exostoses, as a rule, do not manifest until after puberty, usually at about 19 years of age. They grow slowly and progressively until they reach a certain size, and then they remain stationary. It is observed in families as an autosomal dominant characteristic. Therefore, males and females are equally affected.

Differential Diagnosis (see pp. 37, 61)

Differential diagnosis could include some bone tumors.

Laboratory Aids

None.

Treatment

Surgical elimination should be undertaken only if the condition causes food to accumulate in the area or when a full-mouth prosthesis is needed.

Torus Palatinus (3E56)

Torus palatinus is an exostosis of the maxilla that is present in the midline of the hard palate. Torus palatinus is inherited as an autosomal dominant condition. X-linked inheritance is suggested by some family pedigrees.

Clinical Features

This exostosis is always present in the palatal midline. It may vary greatly in size from a small, almost imperceptible exostosis to a large, bony mass, occasionally occupying almost all of the hard palate. The lesion does not manifest clinically until after 18 or 19 years of age. It begins growing very slowly until it reaches its maximum size at about 25 years of age, and then it stabilizes in size for life. Torus palatinus is seen with a female-to-male ratio of 2 to 1. It is most frequently found in Eskimos and is least likely in American blacks. Histologically, it consists of mature normal bone.

Differential Diagnosis (see p. 38)

The condition is clinically so typical that a differential diagnosis is not required. Nevertheless, one could include other tumors of bone as well as a displaced salivary gland neoplasm of the palate.

Laboratory Aids

None.

Treatment

Surgical excision is indicated if the torus interferes with phonation or if a full maxillary prosthesis needs to be constructed.

Traumatic Bone Cyst (5B18)

This entity, which is also known by the name of solitary bone cyst or hemorrhagic bone cyst, is a radiolucency generally observed in the body of the mandible. It is most likely produced by intrabony hemorrhage following trauma.

Clinical Features

The cyst is generally asymptomatic and is discovered on routine radiologic examination. It rarely produces facial asymmetry. It is seen with greatest frequency among male patients under 20 years of age. The most frequent location is the mandibular body, but other sites, such as the chin and maxillary bone, can be affected. The teeth in the area are always vital. Radiologically it can be described as a radiolucency of variable size that does not displace teeth and does not destroy the cortical plates. This radiolucency has a tendency to extend in between the roots of the neighboring teeth and in between the teeth with a typical dome-shaped appearance. It does not produce root resorption.

Differential Diagnosis (see p. 59)

A great variety of lesions can be included in the differential diagnosis, with odontogenic tumors, giant cell granuloma of the jaws, fibrous dysplasia, and odontogenic keratocyst being the most likely.

Laboratory Aids

If biopsy of the lesion is undertaken, a lack of epithelial lining will be observed.

Treatment

The treatment is usually surgical. Upon opening, as a rule, the cavity either is empty or contains some uncoagulated blood. Repair is achieved in a short period of time after surgical opening.

Tuberculous Lymphadenitis (1D47; 1E49)

Tuberculous lymphadenitis is an infection of the cervical lymph nodes by the tubercle bacillae (*Mycobacterium tuberculosis*), which are thought to gain access through the oral tissues or the tonsils and then to produce tubercle granulomas within the lymph nodes. Exposure to milk from infected cows is a possible source of infection. Caseation and discharge of the contents of the tubercle through sinuses in the neck was termed scrofula. Today, tuberculosis tends to be found in persons in lower socioeconomic levels or in persons with primary or secondary deficiencies of the immune system.

Clinical Features

Several lymph nodes may increase in size at one time and are initially well circumscribed and movable (as in 1E49) but later become fixed by secondary fibrosis. The nodes can be painless, tender, or even painful, and not infrequently they will show inflammation of the covering and surrounding skin. The classic description is that of a painless node that develops a pliable consistency as caseation progresses. The caseous material of the so-called cold abscess will drain to the skin by multiple sinuses that become puckered and bound down by scar tissue (as in 1D47).

Differential Diagnosis (see p. 11)

Lymph nodal pathology of the neck, including infectious mononucleosis, Hodgkin's disease, and metastasis should be considered.

Laboratory Aids

Mantoux testing and smear and culture of the sinus discharge are indicated.

Treatment

Treatment of tuberculosis is in the hands of the physician and generally consists of a combined treatment with isoniazid, streptomycin, and p-aminosalicylic acid. Eight to 12 months may be necessary in some cases for proper treatment. Surgical correction of scrofula reduces the morbidity and shortens the medication period.

Turner's Tooth (4A9, 4B20)

Turner's tooth is characterized by a localized area of enamel hypoplasia generally observed in permanent teeth that replace primary teeth.

Clinical Features

The degree of clinical involvement in this condition is quite variable, ranging from a very minute area of localized enamel hypoplasia to a very large destruction of enamel with or without pigmentation. This condition occurs only in those teeth that replace primary teeth. The etiology has been ascribed to a periapical process in the primary teeth that interferes with proper enamel formation in the permanent tooth germ. One might also consider the probability that this periapical process produces a resorption of already formed tissues in the permanent tooth bud. Due to the position of the permanent tooth bud lingual to the primary teeth, this lesion can be seen only on the buccal surface of these teeth.

Differential Diagnosis (see pp. 47, 48)

Differential diagnosis should include early caries, arrested caries, and enamel hypoplasias of other etiology.

Laboratory Aids

None.

Treatment

In cases of extensive destruction, operative dentistry procedures and/or jacket crowns are indicated.

Ulceration, Traumatic (1B23; 2C33; 2D37; 2E50)

Traumatic ulcers in the oral cavity can be produced by ill-fitting dentures, rough-edged carious teeth, toothbrushing, and dry cotton rolls applied and stripped off during dental procedures. Biting, which often occurs during local anesthesia (as in 1B23), can be particularly traumatic. Traumatic ulcers secondary to suckling may occur on the tongue (as in 2E50), on the lingual frenulum (Riga-Fede's disease), or on the palate.

Clinical Features

Ulcers are found most frequently on the tongue, lips and buccal mucosa. They may be single or multiple. Accompanying symptoms are a burning sensation and pain, especially when eating. A white pseudomembrane may cover the ulcer (as in 2D37). When ulceration is associated with a denture, it usually appears 1 to 2 days after placement of the new prosthesis. Most traumatic ulcers have a rapid and uneventful course of about a week. However, some nonspecific chronic ulcers in older people may persist longer.

Differential Diagnosis (see pp. 10, 23, 24, 25)

Recurrent aphthous ulcer, cyclic neutropenia, and herpetic lesions should be considered. In older patients, squamous cell carcinoma must be ruled out.

Laboratory Aids

None.

Treatment

None. The etiologic trauma should be eliminated. Palliative treatment with local anesthetic creams is indicated to diminish pain especially during mastication.

Verruca Vulgaris (1D41)

Verruca vulgaris (wart) is a benign epithelial hyperplastic response to a virus of the papovavirus group.

Clinical Features

Warts appear either as flesh-colored, frequently multiple, small hyperplastic papules or as a papillary growth composed of multiple white, fingerlike projections (filiform warts). They are commoner in childhood and adolescence, being transmitted apparently by direct contact. Autoinoculation from peripheral sites may occur. Such warts rarely occur in the oral cavity. When they do, they most likely develop in the junction of the vermilion border with the skin. Condyloma acuminatum (venereal warts) has been reported in the oral cavity.

The course and prognosis of verrucae vary; some resolve within a few months, whereas others persist for a period of a year or so. Eventually, they tend to regress spontaneously.

Differential Diagnosis (see p. 11)

Warts should be differentiated from papillomas. If the patient is an adult, lesions such as cutaneous horn, keratoacanthoma, and even early verrucous squamous cell carcinoma should be considered in the differential diagnosis.

Laboratory Aids

If the lesion is biopsied, inclusion bodies and marked proliferation of the granular cell layer will be seen.

Treatment

Keratinolytic materials such as linseed oil, acids (e.g., 12% salicylic acid), and podophyllin (a 25% solution in benzoin) may be used.

Vitamin B^{12} Deficiency (2E55)

Vitamin B^{12} deficiency is the result of the failure of the intestine to absorb the vitamin owing to a lack of intrinsic factor. Intrinsic factor may be absent secondary to surgery of the stomach, as the result of an autoimmune process, or even as a congenital defect. In the last case, the clinical manifestations will be observed during infancy or childhood. Other causes for lack of absorption of vitamin B^{12} are severe gastritis, dietary deficiency, and parasitic or bacterial infections. The hematological manifestation of vitamin B^{12} deficiency is a macrocytic anemia (pernicious anemia). Pernicious anemia shows a familial incidence.

Clinical Features

Glossitis as a consequence of the nutritional and neurological disturbances is the most frequent oral finding in this condition. Oral symptoms may precede the development of hematological findings. A sore, burning sensation in the tongue may persist for several weeks with periods of remission. The tongue is initially pale, with slight flattening of the marginal papillae (as in 2E55); however, with further atrophy of the papillae the tongue becomes smooth and beefy red. Other areas of the oral mucosa may become affected by a peripheral neuritis; angular cheilosis also may be present. Systemic findings include weakness, tingling and numbness of the extremities, difficulty in walking, and even mental disturbances.

Differential Diagnosis (see p. 25)

Deficiencies of the other B vitamins may give similar presentations, and combined deficiencies are usually present.

Laboratory Aids

Blood smears and bone marrow aspirates are examined for cytological changes of pernicicous anemia. Buccal smears may show enlargement and aberration of the nuclei of epithelial cells owing to delayed DNA synthesis. Gastric achlorhydria is a definite requisite to confirm that the lack of vitamin B^{12} is related to pernicious anemia since there are other causes of vitamin B^{12} deficiency.

Treatment

Oral changes are good indicators of improvement after specific therapy.

Wegener's Granulomatosis (3B14)

Wegener's granulomatosis is a systemic vasculitis, probably of autoimmune etiology.

Clinical Features

This disease affects both sexes equally, most frequently individuals in the third or fourth decade of life. The oral lesions, when present, manifest on the gingiva as multiple erythematous granular enlargements of the marginal and attached gingiva resembling pyogenic granulomas (as in 3B14). Granular and ulcerative lesions may also be present on the lips and the oral soft tissues. Ecchymosis may be present. An oroantral fistula may develop.

Lung involvement accounts for the persistent cough, and kidney disease may give flank pain. Renal failure and cerebrovascular accidents may result in death.

Differential Diagnosis (see p. 36)

The oral differential diagnosis should include diphenylhydantoin hyperplasia, gingival fibromatosis of various etiologies and multiple pyogenic granulomas. In some cases malignant lymphoma might also be considered.

Laboratory Aids

Biopsy demonstrates necrotizing vasculitis and multinucleated giant cells.

Treatment

The disease was formerly highly fatal with a survival rate of a year or less. Today, cytotoxic drugs (i.e., cyclophosphamides) achieve total remission in the majority of cases.

White Sponge Nevus (2B18)

White sponge nevus, or Cannon's disease, is an autosomal dominant, benign dyskeratosis of the epithelium of mucous membranes resulting from a disorder of tonofibrils.

Clinical Features

This disorder is congenital in some instances and develops during adolescence in others. The buccal, gingival, and lingual mucosae and the mucosa of the floor of the mouth are affected by a corrugated, spongy whitening that may be folded or finely papillated. The vaginal, labial, anal, rectal, and nasal mucosae may also be affected. The condition persists unchanged with no complications.

Differential Diagnosis (see p. 22)

Hereditary benign intraepithelial dyskeratosis, pachyonychia congenita, and Darier-White's disease should be distinguished. Leukoedema and pseudomembranous candidiasis should also be considered.

Laboratory Aids

Buccal smears will show paranuclear and perinuclear condensations of cytoplasm that, under electron microscopy, are found to be tonofibrils. Biopsy will demonstrate marked spongiosis of the oral epithelium.

Treatment

None.

INDEX

Index

Boldface numbers refer to Patient Histories; those in regular type refer to pages in this atlas.